About the authors

Mary and Linda are both internationally recognised pioneers in the anti-diet movement.

MARY EVANS YOUNG

Mary is a staff development consultant, specializing in women's issues. Because of her own experience and from working with hundreds of women she is aware of the destructive effect of negative body image and yo-yo dieting on women's confidence and self esteem.

Following the suicide of a size 14 teenager who felt she was too fat, Mary started Diet Breakers to help women recover from the tyranny of thinness through her Taming The Diet Dragon workshops. Mary is the originator of International No Diet Day which is celebrated on 6th May each year. She lives in Oxfordshire.

LINDA OMICHINSKI

Linda is a registered dietician and accredited fitness leader with twenty years nutritional experience including private counselling and working in diabetic and cardiovascular clinics.

Struck by the large number of her patients who lost weight only to regain it shortly afterwards, Linda decided a new approach was called for. She has used her professional experience and the latest research to develop the innovative *You Count, Calories Don't* programme for better health. Linda lives in Manitoba and is the Canadian Co-ordinator for International No Diet Day.

Also by Mary Evans Young

Diet Breaking, having it all without having to diet

Also by Linda Omichinski

Tailoring Your Tastes

YOU COUNT, CALORIES DON'T

Linda Omichinski,
with Mary Evans Young

Hodder & Stoughton

First published in Canada in 1992 by Tamos Books Inc.
First published in Great Britain in 1996 by Hodder & Stoughton
A division of Hodder Headline PLC

10 9 8 7 6 5 4 3 2 1

Illustrations by Sandra Storen

British Library Cataloguing in Publication Data

Omichinski, Linda
You Count, Calories Don't
I. Title   II. Young, Mary Evans
613.2

ISBN 0 340 65443 0

Typeset by Hewer Text Composition Services, Edinburgh
Printed and bound in Great Britain by
Mackays of Chatham PLC

Hodder and Stoughton Ltd
A Division of Hodder Headline PLC
338 Euston Road
London NW1 3BH

Dedication

In appreciation of all those working in the anti-diet movement to genuinely improve the health and well being of people around the world.

Contents

'An important part of the *You Count, Calories Don't* approach is teaching people to accept themselves as they are. It's a concept that focuses on a healthy lifestyle rather than dieting and calories.'

Alice Krueger, Food Editor

'As a nutrition and lifestyle counsellor, I know that diets don't work. Instead, I use *You Count, Calories Don't*! The innovative ideas and proven techniques described in this book empower clients toward a healthier, and happier, approach to food and life.'

Kathleen Harrison, M.Sc., R.D.,
Community Nutrition Consulting

'People are so preoccupied with weight and cholesterol as health risk factors they ignore the importance of a healthy lifestyle. Without this focus, control of weight and cholesterol usually fail. *You Count, Calories Don't* offers a common sense approach to establishing and *maintaining* a healthier way of life.'

Bob McGregor, M.D.

'Inside every body shape there is a person of worth who can achieve pleasure and satisfaction from his or her own abilities. Ideal weights are individual. The advice in *You Count, Calories Don't* enables the reader to be free of the diet mentality and embrace positive day-to-day changes that promote healthful living and a sense of wellbeing.'

Dr Rena Mendelson, Director, School of Nutrition

'I was so busy with my family's needs I rarely took time for myself or considered what I wanted from life. *You Count, Calories Don't* was instrumental in making me realise the importance of having goals for myself too. The programme helped me get out of the diet mentality and make some important changes in my life which will reflect on my family's future.'

Maureen MacKay, programme participant

Foreword
By Mary Evans Young

Stopping dieting, for me, was a sort of rebellion. I had had enough. I knew diets didn't make me permanently thin, ecstatically happy or more successful. In fact I knew in my bones that dieting was not good for me – or anybody come to that.

I had trained as a psychotherapist for six years and had been in personal therapy too, so I had many insights into my personal issues around eating and weight, but I had not completely managed to translate that awareness to food. After all, what do you eat when you stop dieting? Most of us have been confused into thinking a weight loss diet and a healthy diet are the same thing. Weight loss organisations call their regimes 'healthy eating plans'. But don't be confused. Their names usually give them away and their advertisements always do. A healthy, well balanced diet is really only possible when we relax around food. How can we relax around food if the object of eating is to change ourselves because we are encouraged to feel we are not good enough? Of course, we can't. So we develop concepts of good and bad food and think in terms of 'oughts', 'shoulds' and 'mustn'ts'.

Time and again journalists who come to interview me are under the impression that to stop counting calories automatically means stuffing yourself stupid with cream doughnuts. Part of the problem is that the diet mentality has gripped most of us – individually and collectively. When I appeared on *The Krystal Rose Show* with Professor Tom Sanders and Alice Mahon MP to discuss International No Diet Day, a trolley loaded with cream cakes was wheeled on to the set at the end of the show for the audience to 'celebrate' the day. Tom and I were about the only people who did not take a cake. I looked at them, but there was nothing I fancied. Tom said, 'I might have had a piece of apple tart if there'd been any.'

Another example of the diet mentality is people's belief that

You Count, Calories Don't

those who do not diet are always fat. Not true. Tom Sanders
isn't fat. Linda Omichinski isn't fat. I believe it ought to be
irrelevant whether a person is fat or thin. The most important
things, surely, are health and happiness. However, in these size-
obsessed days I know that many people are terrified of becoming fat. I am against discrimination on the basis of size (or
anything else for that matter), and I know a person can be fit
and fat. During the three years that I have been living the *You
Count, Calories Don't* (YCCD) philosophy I am slowly but
surely returning to my natural weight. I don't know how much I
weigh because I don't weigh myself any more. I am not a thin
woman and I am not a fat woman. I am my own woman, which
is the most comfortable and natural size I have been since before
I started dieting at the age of twelve.

Participants on my Taming the Diet Dragon workshops (previously called Do You Really Need to Diet?) who had started
feeling good about themselves through building self-esteem and
positive body image, wanted something more. There comes a
time when, having made peace with food, you start wanting to
eat healthily to increase your chances of living to a ripe old age.
And, if we are parents, we want to help our children avoid the
pernicious diet trap and live healthy active lives, too.

I came across Linda Omichinski's work when I was in
America. She came well recommended: she is a leading pioneer
in the 'non-diet approach health professionals' circle in America
and in her native Canada. Nevertheless, at first glance I had my
doubts that her plan would be able to do all that she suggests.
Linda, after all, is a Registered Dietitian, not a reformed dieter.
She has never been a dieter, so how could she know what it's
like? Her answer to this is that non-dieters generally have a
healthier approach to food and eating and that dieters can learn
from them. I agree with her: we non-dieters do have a healthier
approach to food, eating, weight and life in general, **and if you
follow the advice in this book, so will you.**

Anyway, believing that developing a healthy eating pattern
would be damned hard, I decided to try out her suggestions for
myself before taking things any further. As she suggested, I
started gradually to embrace the philosophy of the programme
which, incidentally, is called HUGS in Canada and elsewhere.

I believe in the set point theory – that we all have a natural weight that our bodies fight to defend. *You Count, Calories Don't* is not about weight loss and it is not a diet. Unlike most diets, this programme is liberating. It starts with the premise that you are of value and are worth taking care of – right now, not when you have lost weight. It shows you how to develop a healthier eating pattern that will last you a lifetime.

Personally, I have moved from being a person who thought about food twenty-five hours a day (as I ate breakfast I was thinking about lunch) to someone who eats, forgets about food and is able to get on with my day-to-day life in peace. The approach is simple, so simple that you may think you're not doing it at first, and that is why it works. For someone who has done a lot of dieting (the old edicts 'if it ain't hurting, it ain't working' and 'no pain, no gain' sink in deep) this may take a bit of time to get used to. Unlike weight loss diets, this plan teaches you how to trust your body and get back in touch with your natural feelings of hunger and fullness, rather than depending on diet sheets and other external factors.

As a dieter I did not trust my body. I imagined that if I ate what I really wanted I would be out of control, but I have discovered that my body can and does tell me what to eat, and when to stop. I simply had not given it a chance. And guess what? I don't want to eat cream doughnuts and chocolate all the time. In fact, I don't much like doughnuts: they have about as much appeal as an egg sandwich.

The *You Count, Calories Don't* approach has also transformed my attitude towards physical activity. Learning to do it for pleasure rather than pain has given me a genuine liking for exercise which would never have seemed possible when I was exercising solely to lose weight. For the first time in my life I actually enjoy physical activity – not the knees bend, arms stretch stuff, but gentle activity.

Of course, this book is not a magic solution. There are no magic solutions, but this book can help you change your mindset and your approach to yourself from a negative diet mentality to one of support and appreciation. It is a step-by-step health plan, developed by a qualified health professional, which is gaining recognition worldwide and has received very favourable results in a recent research study in the *Journal of the Canadian Dietetic Association.** It has been shown to have helped a wide range of people: diabetics, compulsive dieters, people with weight concerns, recovered eating disorder sufferers, ex-smokers, women with pre-menstrual syndrome (PMS), and people who are simply interested in healthier eating and living. It is regularly recommended by doctors, dietitians, nurses, counsellors and therapists who are looking for more than just another diet sheet to help their patients and clients regain control of their eating weight and their life. *You Count, Calories Don't* (YCCD) is being introduced by many personnel officers and human resources development professionals because they recognise the benefits of a healthy workforce and the damage done by the diet mentality to both staff and the organisation.

As you work your way through the book you'll notice the repetition of key points. This reinforcement is deliberate: the diet mentality can become ingrained and hard to shift. Approach the plan at a comfortable pace. The action points at the end of each chapter are there to provide a practical focus for change. You'll achieve some more easily than others. So be prepared to return to those that require more time to integrate into your new lifestyle. Remember, there is no rush. **This programme is for life!**

I know from my personal experience from talking to the Diet Breakers Facilitators who run the YCCD ten-week programme around the British Isles, and from programme participants themselves, that learning to eat and live well is the foundation to looking after and nurturing all aspects of yourself and fulfilling your potential. Here is what three of our participants told a journalist from the *Sunday Telegraph*:

Liz Sokoski, 41, PR Consultant and now a Diet Breakers Facilitator

'I did them all – Scarsdale, Mayo, Hay, slimming clubs. My weight fluctuated from eight to ten stone. When I got down to

---

* *Journal of the Canadian Dietetic Association*, summer issue (vol 56, no. 2) 1995 entitled 'Reduction of Dieting Attitudes and Practises after Participation in a Non-Diet Lifestyle Program'.

eight stone people said, "You look fantastic!" But I had to spend all my time maintaining that level because it wasn't my true weight. I was never really happy. When you're totally focused on food, you put your life on hold. I'd say to myself I couldn't do certain things until I could fit into a size 12 dress. In between diets I went up to eleven and a half stone because I couldn't recognise my body's hunger signals. Now, through not dieting and returning to normal eating, I've lost over a stone in five months. I'm very happy. I'm much more creative and spontaneous. I'm my real self, not the person I was pretending to be for all those years.'

Di Smith, 25, Secretary in bank share dealing service

'I was totally addicted. I spent thousands of pounds on slimming pills, books, drinks and powders. For one year, I lived on nothing but liquid diets. My life was absolute hell. Whatever I was doing, I was thinking about food. My relationship failed; I even missed an opportunity for promotion because I was too tired to cope. I was so out of touch with my appetite I didn't know how to eat. It took a lot of therapy and counselling to get me off the diets. Three months ago I heard about Diet Breakers and wished I'd known about them earlier. Now I no longer have mood swings or cravings. If I'm not hungry I don't eat. If I fancy a cake I have one. I never count calories. I'm eight stone and happy. I look back and think what a waste.'

Poppy Szaybo, 25, Freelance photographer

'I put on weight at puberty. I lost confidence, got used to being overweight and put on more. I tried to diet and went to Weight Watchers, but because I was taking away the things I wanted to eat, I'd binge. It affected every aspect of my life. I'd never go on a beach, never go to night clubs and turned down jobs because I was not happy with myself. Going to Diet Breakers was hard. I'm seen as a very confident person in my work, but I've always been terrified of exposing myself. Being in a group with others who had a weight problem helped. Now I eat what I want and stop when I'm full. I no longer have cravings for sugary things because I don't deprive myself of them. In fact, I don't have that much of an appetite. I can see I've lost weight but I don't know how much. That's not the point; happiness is not determined by the scales but by how you feel, and for the first time in my life I really like myself. It's such a relief.'

Editing this book has been a labour of love. I want to enable as many people as possible to embrace this concept because we'll all be a lot healthier and happier and can then get on with the things in life that really do count.

Mary Evans Young
Oxfordshire, England
Summer 1995

Foreword
To Canadian Edition

For the last two decades, in an effort to look good and feel great, North Americans have been caught up in a continuous cycle of weight loss and weight gain. Many people lose weight; however, few maintain their slimmer figures. Almost no one feels great in the up and down weight loss/weight gain process. It seems reasonable to assume that if every weight control product or programme on the market could provide the fast, permanent weight loss they promise, the diet industry would have gone out of business years ago. Instead, diet regimes flourish, and countless individuals literally starve themselves for months to lose a few pounds, only to regain some, all, or more weight as soon as the diet is stopped. The disappointment and loss of self-worth take an emotional toll on the victims of these unrealistic promises. To make matters worse, the focus on 'diet' and 'thin' seems to have spawned an epidemic of such eating disorders as anorexia nervosa and bulimia which often begin as a simple effort to lose a few pounds. Clearly, the programmes and products that are designed to promote rapid weight loss do not offer permanent help and because of this, people who follow these diets neither look good nor feel great in the long term.

Perhaps we are placing the emphasis on the wrong aspect. All of our scientific evidence suggests that ideal weights are individual and that maintaining the weight that is right for you contributes to better looks and better health. This approach is founded on two important concepts. First, we must recognise that we cannot all expect to look like the thin models we see in magazines and films. Second, each of us can be individually attractive and vibrant through a healthy lifestyle which includes a balance of regular, enjoyable exercise and healthy tasty food choices. This is the best way to look good and feel great!

In the following pages, Linda Omichinski tells us how to achieve this goal. She has utilised all the most up-to-date scientific theories on energy metabolism and food behaviour and put into practice a set of activities designed to enhance physical and emotional health. In a clear and practical way, she helps each reader to recognise that inside every body shape there is a person of worth who can achieve pleasure and satisfaction from their own abilities. Ms Omichinski's advice enables each reader to escape from the trap of inflated promises and unfulfilled desires and to embrace the positive day-to-day changes that promote healthy living and a sense of well-being.

The advice is excellent. This book should be read over and over again until the principles are gradually integrated into a lifestyle change for a better, healthier you.

Rena A. Mendelson, M.S., D.Sc.
Director
Professor of Nutrition
School of Nutrition, Consumer
and Family Studies
Ryerson Polytechnical Institute
Toronto, Canada

Preface

The You Count, Calories Don't Programme is for Everyone

Western society is obsessed with being slim. It is a cultural fad that totally ignores the importance of healthy living. Unfortunately, this preoccupation with diet can be transmitted to others. A recent study indicated that two out of three mothers who thought they weighed too much (even when they didn't) passed this anxiety on to their daughters, who became chronically unhappy with their weight.[1]

Although diets seem to have increased people's consciousness about weight and food, they have not made people healthier. Research proves that diet and exercise regimes that focus on weight loss as the goal are seldom successful in the long term, which leaves the person feeling discouraged and less in control of their own body.[2,3] More people are becoming fed up with dieting and are seeking an alternative that will work with their bodies, not against them.[4]

As a consulting dietitian in hospitals and with private clients, I am continually concerned about my clients' food and weight problems. Initially, I used the traditional approach of designing individualised diets for clients whom I saw for weight control, diabetes, risk factors for heart disease, and other health reasons.

Of course in the short term, diets did work. Weight loss and modified eating habits were always evident. Following my prescribed diet for them, clients returned to report their successes and this led me to believe that this approach was valid.

Yet on follow-up a few years later the results were disappointing. In many cases, clients were worse off in terms of health than when they first came to see me. Unfortunately, health professionals tend to blame the client for the failure. Diets after all do work, if you follow the strict regime.

As I continued to observe this weight loss/weight gain cycle, however, I began to question the traditional approach. Following the medical model I had learned seemed to work only in the short term. I searched through the scientific literature to find answers, but found them instead by questioning my clients. It was through studying the needs of my clients and listening to their concerns that this lifestyle programme emphasising a non-dieting approach to healthy living came into existence.

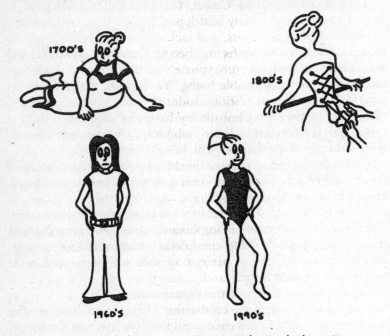

'When did this preoccupation with weight begin?'

This book is based on the HUGS programme that I established and tested in the community over the past eight years. It has provided high client satisfaction. The process is satisfying and fun to do, and it works! It can help you to be the best that you can be.

You Count, Calories Don't focuses on the importance of building a sense of mastery or control over your life which helps build self-esteem. Empowerment to do this is skill-based and is accomplished in a step-by-step manner. As one skill is mastered, the next skill is introduced while still reinforcing the skill already learned.

This skill-building process involves changing your thinking and gradually fine-tuning your lifestyle in order to enjoy healthy living. **The focus is on the process, not on a quick end result.** The journey is designed to be pleasurable so that it can be continued and the results can be permanent.

To achieve this, *You Count, Calories Don't* addresses the underlying causes of many health problems. These are poor self-esteem and lifestyle habits, and lack of confidence. By realising that *you count*, and by feeling better about yourself, you will want to take time to nurture yourself through healthy enjoyable eating and active enjoyable living. *You Count, Calories Don't* provides a health promotion model that allows the individual the freedom to take responsibility for their own health.

Anyone who has ever dieted, whether for a particular health reason or for weight loss, will benefit from this book. This alternative concept focuses on health and wellbeing and shows how to put food and activity into a healthy perspective that is comfortable to continue for life.

The lifestyle you choose is important. Unhealthy lifestyles can cause such life-threatening conditions as heart disease, cancer, and strokes. Yet eighty percent of lifestyle diseases can be prevented. By recognising and reducing health risks, a person can start making wellness the preferred lifestyle.

This book emphasises celebrating and enjoying food, not depriving yourself. Everyone can do this by acquiring a taste for less sweet, less fattening foods which will lead to choosing different foods as tastes change.

This approach is for everyone, and it does work. Even for individuals with diabetes you ask? The answer is yes. I remember instructing clients on a diabetic diet and then when they got complications (i.e. high-cholesterol levels), instructing them on a low-cholesterol diet. The clients became confused and frustrated and I thought there must be a simpler way that would provide a unified approach. This programme was my answer.

The first chapter shows how this programme coincides with the principles and recommendations of the Diabetes Association, Heart Foundation, Dietetic Association, and Cancer

Foundation, as well as addressing the issue of obesity. All of these programmes emphasise eating more high-fibre foods (carbohydrates) for immediate energy, some protein for sustained energy, and gradually decreasing fat intake.

The difference in the programme is the approach. Most special diets are based on 'dos' and 'don'ts'. Eat only thirty percent of your calories from fat. Watch your weight. Increase your activity. These are necessary, but they miss the point by focusing on giving instructions to follow rather than empowering the individual to want to make healthier choices. *You Count, Calories Don't* shows you a simple and effective way to healthy living!

The concepts presented in this book integrate three positive life choices: enjoyable, healthy eating; enjoyable, physical activity; and positive self-image and body image. *You Count, Calories Don't* shows you how to integrate these components of wellbeing and quality of life into your everyday lifestyle so that you too can feel better about yourself.

Many clients are hesitant about exercise because of negative feelings about physical activity. This book shows you how to be aware of your body's needs in order to eat and exercise for energy and enjoyment! It shows you how to restore balance to your life in order to be better prepared for stressful situations. In fact, you will see how you can make stress work for you.

This refreshing approach is welcomed enthusiastically by health professionals. Yet many counsellors are hesitant to try the method since it is new and unfamiliar and different from professional training. My recommendation to health professionals is to introduce the method gradually. With this step-by-step process as a guide, you can begin to focus on health indicators rather than numbers on the scale as the new measure of success.

If people focus on wellness and learn to help themselves to achieve their potential for spiritual, mental, social, and physical wellbeing, they will get on the road to healthy living. This guide takes a holistic approach and can be used to accompany individuals or group counselling.

Introduction

To *You* Count, *Calories Don't*

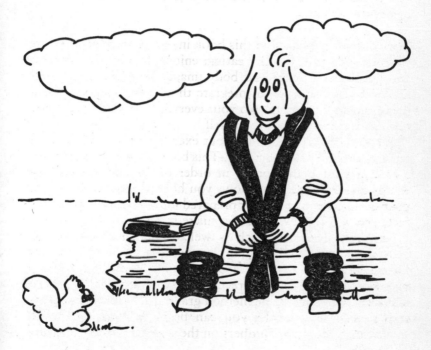

This programme is an alternative to dieting. It allows you to regain control of your weight, food and life by presenting a positive approach to healthy living and by helping you to feel better about yourself.

If you recognise yourself here, this programme can help you:

Rush! Rush!
No breakfast. Quick lunch. Dragging by 4 o'clock.
Raiding the fridge before dinner and lunching and munching after dinner until bedtime.
Your eating is out of control.

You're preoccupied with food and weight.
Your life is centred around the 'dos' and 'don'ts' of eating, leading to a round of indulging, guilt, and denial.
If you eat a piece of cake today you'll have to diet tomorrow. You feel you are chained to a diet.
You would like to be 'free' from the chains of dieting and get on with the rest of your life.

You plan to starve during the week to compensate for the anticipated binge at Uncle Joe's wedding next Saturday.
But your willpower runs out and suddenly the biscuit tin is empty.
Your nagging hunger gets the better of you.

> You're on a diet, but overeating on holidays is socially acceptable.
> Your guilt feelings lead to the next diet.
> This on-again off-again dieting leads to the weight loss/weight gain cycle.

> You're a nibbler. You eat food simply because it's there.
> You feel tired and draggy.
> Now you're interested in learning how you can live a healthier lifestyle.

YCCD works on the premise that diets set you up for failure. **Freeing yourself from the diet mentality is the key to regaining control.** We focus on health and wellness rather than on weight and slimness, allowing each person to adjust to their natural weight, which is genetically predetermined. We counter the pervasive cult of ultra slimness in our society. The perfectly proportioned, ultra slim body is an unnatural goal promoted by multimedia advertising. We are conditioned to believe that we must conform and pursue the illusory perfection of slimness. We follow the perfect diet, eat the right way, and allow this pursuit to overtake and control our daily lives.[1] YCCD believes individual differences are to be rejoiced in, not derided.

Through this programme you will learn different ways of looking after yourself, and will acquire the skills, techniques, attitudes and mindset that will allow you to take charge of your life. The inner strength that comes from a feeling of self-worth creates a desire to nurture yourself by taking care of your body and mind. You will find the energy and desire to fine-tune your eating habits and be more active. The sense of accomplishment and the satisfaction gained from increased levels of activity and improved eating will establish the cycle: positive thinking, healthy enjoyable eating and active enjoyable living. You will become a vibrant, attractive person at the weight that is right for your body and you will maintain this new you through the balanced cycle you have established.

BALANCE IN LIFE: Healthy Living

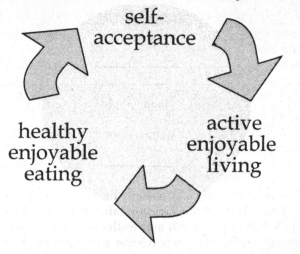

self-
acceptance

healthy
enjoyable
eating

active
enjoyable
living

WHAT TO EXPECT

The programme can help you achieve this balance in life by learning how to face reality in a positive way and empowering yourself with the freedom of choice. It shows you how to respond normally to food, through celebration rather than denial, how to live in the present and focus on the moment at hand, and how to savour it. Success does not mean trying to be someone else or comparing yourself to other people and accepting imposed standards of diet and fitness. It means striving to be the best that you can be with what you have been given genetically rather than aiming for the traditional quick fix of instant weight loss, and disappointment when the weight returns.[2]

The struggle to maintain or reach an unrealistic ideal weight results in people working against their bodies. There is a proper weight for each individual called the set point and this comfortable level becomes the weight focus for healthy living. Society tells us in a hundred subtle ways how we should look and behave. It takes courage and determination to listen to your body, acknowledge the right weight for you and accept yourself as you are. When you do this there is no stress and maintaining the new you becomes easy. One of our top priorities is enjoyment, not struggle.

You Count, Calories Don't is for people who are ready for something more than the usual diet regime and are ready to focus on the more achievable goals of self-acceptance and healthy lifestyle. It is for those who feel dissatisfied with their bodies or out of control around food. It can help people with high cholesterol, diabetes, pre-menstrual syndrome or the new non-smoker. In fact it's suitable for everyone: everyone deserves a healthy lifestyle!

HOW TO USE THIS BOOK

To derive the most benefit from the book, read it slowly one chapter at a time, taking time to digest the information and put the suggestions into action. To assist you we have listed things to work on at the end of each chapter, starting with Chapter 2. You will notice some repetition in the ideas and practical suggestions throughout the book. This is deliberate – to reinforce the learning and help you live it.

There is too much to take on board all at once – especially if you have tried dieting in the past. Much of what is suggested will be different from the traditional all or nothing, quick fix diet mentality. So take your time and read the book over again to help you fine-tune your lifestyle and sustain it gradually to become a happier, healthier person. Tune into the excitement of the ideas presented and look at the examples. This will help make the information real for you. As you proceed step-by-step, try out each suggestion and enjoy the journey to healthy living.

This book has evolved as a written guide to the *You Count, Calories Don't* programme but it can be used by itself or in conjunction with the affirmation tapes or fitness video (see order form at end of book).

Before you continue, take a moment to fill out this lifestyle quiz. As you move through the book, you will notice that your attitudes will change. This is part of the internal quick fix that will set you up to win! As you proceed the process will become easier. Discovering the new inner you gradually changes the outer you. This will be observed and these changes will be permanent. The lifestyle quiz will help to rate your progress in achieving a healthy lifestyle and obtaining a healthier outlook towards life. Your life out of balance will become your life in balance. You will learn how to revitalise yourself by seeing your life as a series of challenges, not as a series of problems.

GETTING THE MOST FROM THIS BOOK

The first step in seeing your life as a series of challenges is to feel in charge. In order to feel in charge you have to make your own choices. Try changing the way you speak and the phrases you use. Think enthusiastically. Use sentences in your subconscious such as:

'I like and respect myself.'
'I am worthy of the respect of others.'
'No matter what anyone says or does, I am a worthwhile person.'

Replace 'have to' with phrases such as:

'I want to,'
'I like to,'
'I choose to,'
'I love to,'
'I believe I can.'

When you approach a task, put your heart in it, go with the flow and experience the power within you that will allow you to develop your inner strengths. Allow the experience of learning about your inner resources to develop, and picture yourself being effective in stressful situations.

- SET YOUR GOAL. Make it realistic. Focus on the attitude and lifestyle changes. Be specific. For example, say to yourself 'I will eat regularly, starting with a balanced breakfast.'
- VISUALISE THE GOAL. Picture yourself in your mind eating regularly as part of your daily routine.

LIFESTYLE QUIZ

1 Always
2 Very often
3 Often
4 Sometimes
5 Rarely
6 Never

☐ I am unhappy with myself the way I am.

☐ I am preoccupied with a desire to be thinner.

☐ I weigh myself several times a week.

☐ I am more concerned with the number on the scale than my overall sense of wellbeing.

☐ I think about burning up calories when I exercise.

☐ I am out of tune with my body for natural signals of hunger and fullness.

☐ I eat for reasons other than physical hunger.

☐ I eat too quickly, not taking time to focus on my meal and to taste, savour, and enjoy my food.

☐ I fail to take time for activities for myself.

☐ I fluctuate between periods of sensible, nutritious eating and out-of-control eating.

☐ I give too much time and thought to food.

☐ I tend to skip meals, especially early in the day, so I can 'save up' my food for one big feast.

☐ I engage in all-or-nothing thinking. I tend to feel that if I can't do it all, or do it well, what's the point?

☐ I try to be all things to all people.

☐ I strive for perfection in my life.

☐ I criticise myself for not achieving my goals.

☐ **Total** Add 4 to the score to determine your percentage.

(Note: Compare this score with same quiz at end of book.)

- AFFIRM THE GOAL. Repeat it in your mind and practise it so that it becomes second nature at the subconscious level.

- LOCK ONTO THE GOAL. Develop a sense of momentum that will move you forward, creating the inner excitement of 'mini-successes' that keep you progressing. Focus! Focus! Focus and take action.

If you feel good about yourself, you don't need to use food as a crutch to make yourself feel better. If you use affirmations to feel better about yourself, you no longer need to turn to food as a temporary comforter. Use the following affirmation to help you put this way of thinking into action.

'I like myself. Therefore I will take care of myself and nurture myself with healthy eating and enjoyable activity. If I feel good about myself, I don't need to turn to food to comfort me.'

LIFESTYLE ADJUSTMENT

'I don't want to make a lifestyle change – I want to follow a diet.' This is what most people say when confronted with this new way of thinking. It's easier just to follow a prescribed regime than take control yourself. But lifestyle change is exciting. Once you've started you won't want to stop. Let's begin by understanding what it means.

Change is always difficult at first, but once you believe that you have the ability to find the right balance of food, activity, and attitudes to life, you can break free from diet sheets and meal plans forever. Once you understand our philosophy, you can put it to work for yourself, leaving room for flexibility.

I think most of us agree that diets don't work. You regain the weight you lost because you go back to your former way of eating and living. When you realise this you no longer blame yourself for the failure of the diet. A change of lifestyle and change of attitude towards food and yourself are what is needed. You need to acquire skills that can be used in every aspect of life. This will result in a healthier you.

Dieting produces results too. But the weight loss achieved after following a rigid diet is usually temporary. The new diet is often too drastic to be maintained, and as soon as you stop following the diet you gain weight again. Because it is an artificial and unpleasant way of eating, a diet is stressful, both physically and emotionally. The diet controls you. You live by the diet sheet. You lose the weight but have you really learned anything about eating or about yourself? Can you realistically eat this way for the rest of your life, depriving yourself, always thinking of food? Is your goal of weight loss realistic and can you possibly reach the goal expected of you? Can you endure until the end of the diet without going off it?

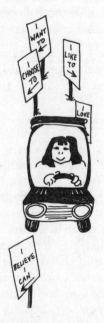

So many of my clients have told me that when they were in weight-loss programmes they would starve themselves before weighing in so they could mark the weight loss in their little book and appear to be successful. When I asked them about activities after a weight-loss meeting, they replied, 'We rewarded ourselves at the cake shop. We were starving!'

Did you ever notice how few people stay for the lecture at many of these weight-loss meetings? All that is important to clients is the number on the scale. This is a negative approach to weight control. It involves cycles of starvation and binging. No new skills are learned and the problem of weight control is never solved.

Actually, the scale, as your measure of success, gives you a false sense of security. A scale focuses solely on results, and causes you to work against your body to achieve this end. Diets follow an external cue. They try to impose change on your behaviour and your way of doing things. This external motivation or 'hype' that occurs at each meeting keeps you going for a while. Eventually you come to rely on the support and can't do without it. There is no motivation from within.

When the weight is lost you feel good because of all the acceptance and compliments you receive. When the compliments stop and the attention is gone, the weight goes back on. You cannot maintain the rigid diet, but you feel ashamed that you lack the willpower. Your sense of self-worth diminishes and you begin to equate slimness with self-confidence. You lose sight of who you are. That poses a critical question. Are you losing weight for society's approval or for yourself?

Then you diet again to punish yourself for not looking the way society dictates that you should look. Then you binge to rebel against dieting and society's refusal to accept different body shapes. Up and down you go, along with your sense of self-worth and self-esteem.

In contrast to this, lifestyle changes are gradual because they are a learning process. Step-by-step adjustments allow your body to embrace the newness. This does not mean going from fried potatoes to brown rice all in one swoop. Your body would be likely to rebel by craving sugar, because the change was too sudden to allow your body to adjust. A more realistic approach would be to gradually introduce white rice, possibly once a week, then with time, mix white rice with brown rice, and only a year later would you have brown rice more frequently.

Lifestyle changes are positive and enjoyable. As your body adjusts it doesn't rebel. You can live with it and you feel a sense of accomplishment. Stress also diminishes when you are not competing against others, but rather looking within yourself to find your own level of progress. The focus is on the process, the facts, the skills, and the techniques. These are the 'how-tos' of living a healthy lifestyle. You are not controlled by your diet.

Rather you are empowered to effect change and take back control.

The motivation for change comes from within as you proceed towards a new you. You can make changes simply because it makes you feel good and gives you more energy. This programme supports you to accept yourself as you are, the first step in increasing control and improving your self-esteem. Choose to change your lifestyle for yourself, not for anyone else. With more confidence you will not depend on compliments from others to continue to practise your new lifestyle.

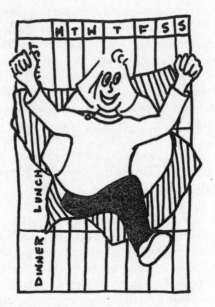

Working with lifestyle change can breathe new excitement into your life. It is a totally positive experience that allows you to eat again, taste, savour, and enjoy food without starving and binging. It puts carbohydrates back into your meals, leaving you satisfied, happy, clear-headed, and in charge. *You count, calories don't.* By focusing on yourself and your needs, learning to tune into and be aware of your body, you will feel better about yourself and your energy level will improve. If you feel better about yourself you will gain confidence in your ability to focus on mini-changes as measures of success.

You don't need to count calories. You need to change your attitude. You don't need self-control for denial, you just need to think normally. You will learn to look at your eating as part of your life. You will be given the tools to deal with the problems as they arise. If you believe you can do it, you can.

1

A Unified Approach for Everyone

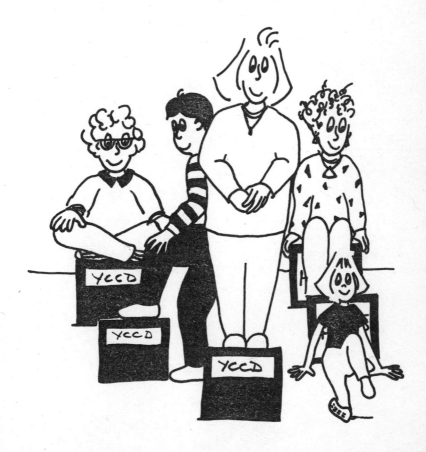

Refer to the section that describes your situation or area of interest. It will provide you with a focus to make the book work best for your needs.

THE PROBLEM	WHAT YCCD CAN DO FOR YOU
Weight concerns	Adopt regular eating habits with lower fat content, increase physical activity, adopt a healthier attitude towards food and activity.
Pre-menstrual syndrome (PMS)	Reduce blood sugar swings that bring on symptoms of PMS. Achieve a balance in eating, physical activity, and decrease caffeine intake to relieve PMS symptoms.
Next generation	Principles that apply to adults can be transferred to children. Getting them away from the diet mentality and helping them accept themselves nurtures an environment conducive to improved self-esteem and a healthier lifestyle.
New non-smoker	Reduce sugar and fat cravings and the urge to smoke by making a lifestyle change and eating in a way that helps to reduce blood sugar swings.
High cholesterol	Adopt regular eating habits with lower fat content, increase physical activity to help reduce the chance of heart disease.
People with diabetes	Balance carbohydrate and protein to stabilise blood sugar, address concerns of weight, acquire a taste for less sugary foods.

WEIGHT CONCERNS

'I can't lose weight without a diet. The diet sheet tells me what to do.'

'I'm losing control. Every time I see food, I want it.'

'I see to be able to keep the weight off only if I stay on the diet. I can't imagine being on a diet for the rest of my life.'

If you are concerned about weight and find that food is the centre of your attention, you would probably like to find a way to deal with this. You need new skills and a different mindset to help you take charge. YCCD can help you find out why diet sheets have prevented you from taking responsibility for your own health.

Learning to eat regularly according to your hunger signals will allow you to stabilise your blood sugar level and reduce your craving for sweets. Acquiring a taste for less sugary and fattening foods will help you to make healthier choices because you no longer crave fats and sugar. YCCD will show you how to achieve this.

PRE-MENSTRUAL SYNDROME (PMS)

'The week before my period, I am absolutely driven to eat sweets and junk food. I don't understand it because I usually have a lot of self-control.'

PMS is brought on by high progesterone levels in the body during the second half of the menstrual cycle. High progesterone levels can cause the body's cells to be resistant to insulin. This means that even though there are normal to high levels of glucose in the blood, the glucose is not able to enter the body's cells. This causes cravings for sweets and increased appetite – a roller coaster effect.

- Well-balanced eating helps to avoid pre-menstrual binging. You may be hungry more frequently during this time because the hormone progesterone reduces the amount of glucose your body's cells receive. Binging can produce higher levels of insulin which may increase the cell's resistance to insulin. Then a roller coaster effect may occur where binging can result in increased hunger.

- Eat more carbohydrates that are complex or lower on the glycaemic index (see Chapter 4). Eating sweets or refined sugars may give symptoms of low blood sugar.

- You can stabilise blood sugar swings and reduce symptoms of irritability by a balanced way of eating.

- If you experience pre-menstrual abdominal bloating choose less salty foods.

- If you experience symptoms of anxiety or irritability, choose foods and beverages lower in caffeine content.

- Stay physically active and take regular aerobic activity to increase your sense of wellbeing, decrease fluid retention, and help relieve depression. This lessening of symptoms may be linked to the rise in endorphins during physical activity which have a relaxing effect.

- Be aware that alcohol, a mood-altering drug, can cause depression and feelings of hopelessness.

If these suggestions don't work you may have a relative deficiency of vitamin B6. This is common among oral contraceptive users. Vitamin B6 is involved in the production of serotonin, a brain chemical related to mood. A relative deficiency of B6 results in reduced synthesis of serotonin and a resulting depression.

Note The literature on B6 is controversial at this time. Many articles state that 100 mg of B6 (pyridoxine) taken daily one week prior to the onset of your period is beneficial. However, a recent study indicates that women who take B6 supplements for long periods of time can develop neurological symptoms even with dosages previously thought safe. The minimum dosage that can cause trouble is unknown but is less than the amount commonly prescribed for pre-menstrual tension.[1] The women in this study had taken vitamin B6 in quantities from less than fifty mg to over 200 mg daily for a period of anywhere from six months to over five years. If you are using this supplement, do not use it on a daily basis but only one week prior to the onset of your menstrual period.

Cuing into the enjoyment of exercise is a natural and healthy way to relieve symptoms of depression. Satisfied YCCD clients have related that symptoms of PMS have decreased when they follow our philosophy.

NEXT GENERATION

A mother's constant dieting and discontent with her body often sends messages to the child that they are not okay and need to go on a diet. Our society's preoccupation with perfection, whether it's the 'perfect body' or being the best in school or in sports, can lead a child into a constant struggle to keep up.

Studies indicate that an important factor in adolescent depression and low self-esteem is poor body image. Up to two-thirds of young women between the ages of twelve and twenty-three are unhappy with their weight. The astonishing fact is that most of those who wanted to lose weight were not even overweight. Both boys and girls desire flat abdomens and hard bodies more than they desire health. This fuels the diet industry and produces bestsellers and gimmicks. Ironically, the nation continues to gain weight.[2]

Childhood and adolescence are critical stages in the development of behaviour and attitudes that foster wellbeing and healthy living. Nutrition and exercise habits established in childhood are most likely to persist as an integral part of a person's lifestyle. A sedentary child becomes a sedentary adult. Yet even though parents generally recognise the importance of establishing healthy lifestyle habits, a positive role model can set a good example. Optimal growth, fitness, and feeling good need to be emphasised as goals in order to translate into a healthier lifestyle for the adults of the twenty-first century.[3]

Preschool is the time when parental influence has the greatest impact. If parents foster the attitude that activity is an important part of everyday life, and focus on physical movement rather than sedentary games and watching television, they can encourage children to adopt a healthy lifestyle.

Because of working parents, today's children are more responsible for household duties including food preparation and shopping. They tend to fend for themselves, and eat convenience foods more frequently. Yet sufficient nutrients are vital for the child's health and wellbeing in the growth process. For the adolescent who has limited experience, supervised involvement in food preparation and shopping can help them learn. The focus could be on the immediate benefits of healthy living, such as energy to boost the child's desire for health and wellness.

As parents go through the process of self-discovery by tuning into their bodies for signals of hunger, appropriate levels of activity, time for themselves, and basic needs for happiness, they will notice how these positive attitudes transfer to their children.

Some Suggestions to Consider

- Think twice before asking your child to clean their plate before having dessert or in order to be considered a good child.

- Avoid using food as a reward for good behaviour or to comfort a child when they are not feeling well.

- Try not to establish erratic eating habits where everyone fends for themselves instead of cultivating a special family mealtime.

- Avoid taking the enjoyment out of eating by controlling the child's food intake rather than allowing them to tune into their internal hunger signals for a feeling of fullness.

- Accept the child – don't instill a feeling of not being good enough.

- Think twice before introducing diets as a form of control rather than adopting positive lifestyle habits that become a way of life for the family.

- Avoid centring the focus of holiday occasions on food alone rather than the occasion itself and its meaning, including friendship and conversation as well as the activities of the event.

- Try not to make the child rely on diet products (i.e. diet drinks) that do not allow them to acquire a taste for less sugary foods.

The bonus gained from living a healthy lifestyle is a sense of inner satisfaction when you take responsibility for your own health. It can help to create a better balance in family life.

NEW NON-SMOKER

'I'm afraid to stop smoking because I'll get fat.'

'Smoking helps me keep slim.'

'I need cigarettes to curb my appetite.'

'I'll stop smoking when I've lost thirty pounds.'

Do any of the above statements sound familiar to you? Do you 'jump-start' your body with caffeine and cigarettes, the chemical dynamite that gets you up and running every morning? Can your body survive this torture?

Myths of Smoking and Weight Gain
At first glance Bob looked like a healthy individual. He appeared to be of ideal body weight and was bright and alert. A few weeks later when I walked into his office, the first thing I noticed was the smell of smoke. He told me how he was trying to stop smoking and how he was compelled to have a cigarette. He had been trying to go 'cold turkey' but the withdrawal symptoms were unbearable! Yet he was tired of cigarettes having a hold on his life.

Since Bob was also a heavy coffee drinker, understanding the effect that nicotine and caffeine had on blood sugar levels helped him understand why increased hunger was one of the withdrawal symptoms he was experiencing. Caffeine, like nicotine, can temporarily mask hunger feelings by stimulating the body to release more glucose from its stores in the bloodstream. After our discussion, he decided to gradually wean himself off cigarettes to minimise withdrawal symptoms. At the same time, he would start eating more regularly to combat the increased hunger cravings, and use the appropriate balance of foods to sustain his energy level.

Was that cigarette really necessary after the meal or was it purely habit, to be used as a reward? Could the renewed taste in the food itself be satisfying on its own as he learned to taste and savour his meal? These were some of the questions that he was answering in his own mind.

Smoking is widely used as a technique to control weight. Female smokers are more apt to use smoking to avoid weight gain. Women will also return to smoking to curb weight gain and increased appetite. In contrast, men return to smoking because of excessive stress and a craving for cigarettes.[4]

Bob's lifestyle had been unhealthy. He didn't eat breakfast and was proud of it. He had erratic eating habits, and he smoked one pack of cigarettes and drank ten cups of coffee a day. This excessive stimulation made him on edge. His smoking was really more harmful than excess weight. Because of his lifestyle Bob at 130 pounds had the same health risk as a non-smoker weighing 210 to 230 pounds.

To use smoking as a method of weight control is clearly an inappropriate choice. If he continued smoking, Bob's chance of dying before the age of seventy was almost twice as great as that of a large individual who was a non-smoker.[5] See chart p24.

Nicotine increases metabolism (the number of calories you burn at rest) by about ten percent for heavy smokers, but it is not a recommended way to burn up calories to keep weight down.

If you use smoking for weight control, remember that not everyone gains weight once they stop smoking. If you make a lifestyle change, this can reduce the likelihood of gaining weight. The decrease in metabolic rate that occurs can be offset by an increase in physical activity. Exercise for enjoyment in order to make it permanent. Experience the 'high' that comes from activity.

You should know that even if you smoke this won't keep you from becoming obese. Although smokers weigh an average of only about seven pounds less than non-smokers they can gain weight and often put it on in places that seriously affect their health. Smokers tend to accumulate fat around the waist rather than the hips, and this is associated with a greater risk of heart disease, diabetes, and early death.[6] Once you have stopped smoking, dieting to control your weight is not the answer. Dieting has a negative effect on the metabolic rate, bringing it down by fifteen to thirty percent within a twenty-four to forty-eight hour period.[7] On the other hand, the immediate health benefits of lifestyle change will reduce your desire to smoke.

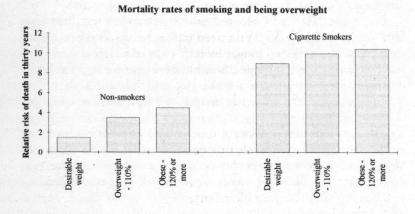

Mortality rates of smoking and being overweight

The secret of successfully stopping smoking and not gaining weight depends on lifestyle change. If you, like Tom, order salad for lunch but spread two packets of salad dressing over it you may as well eat the hamburger your friends are eating. Tom remains hungry, and he is unhappy that he didn't have a hamburger. All he ever talks about is food. His metabolism is being slowed down by his poor eating habits. Since he has been using cigarettes to dampen his appetite he has been out of tune with his natural hunger signals. Now he is using false impressions about healthy eating and denying himself some of the real pleasures of food. Substitution of lower calorie foods (salads) doesn't satisfy unless the person truly enjoys the replacement. Lifestyle change will show Tom how to rev up his metabolism using food and activity.

When you stop smoking, don't diet. Eat sensibly balanced meals that consist of more substance than simply water, vitamins, minerals, and fibre.

Another point to remember is that as a new non-smoker you will get hungry more often because your stomach empties more quickly. Smoking keeps food in your stomach longer so that you can go without food and not feel hungry. When you stop smoking, do not turn to water and diet drinks to help fill you up. You may feel bloated and temporarily full, but this will not keep you going. You need to learn how to eat in a way that keeps you satisfied longer by naturally allowing you to keep food in your stomach longer. Soluble fibre and the right balance in your eating habits can achieve this end.

Some scientists believe that nicotine affects the level of blood sugar (glucose) in the body, so that nicotine withdrawal triggers an increased craving for sweet foods. This may be the result of the lower blood sugar levels that occur when you stop smoking. When your blood sugar levels are low, you feel hungry, especially for something sweet. A balanced lifestyle will show you how to stabilise your blood sugar levels so that those 'highs' and 'lows' level out.

The secretion of insulin pushes glucose (all food is eventually broken down into this simple sugar) into cells to provide energy, thus lowering the blood sugar level and causing hunger. Smoking inhibits insulin secretion causing blood sugar levels to remain higher. This suppresses appetite. Many smokers reach for a cigarette when they are actually physically hungry. Lifestyle change will help you get back in tune with your body. You will learn to eat when you are physically hungry and stop when you are full.

Another disadvantage of smoking is that it cues the end of a meal. At that time you often crave the oral gratification of something sweet. Smokers often turn to a cup of coffee. You will learn the effect that caffeine has on your blood sugar level. Cutting back on coffee will stabilise your blood sugar level and you will begin to rely on food for energy and alertness, rather than on caffeine and cigarettes. You can learn how to break the habit of a cigarette and coffee to end your meal and replace these with healthier options that you will enjoy.

Ask yourself these questions: Do you really want that cigarette or sweet at the end of a meal or is it merely psychologically satisfying? Can it be a habit? If so, you will not feel deprived if you delay smoking the cigarette and confront the urge. Tell yourself that you can have that cigarette later if you still want it.

Breaking the familiar associations and patterns will not give you any anxiety since the real reason you thought you wanted the cigarette is habit, not desire. This is an effective technique for gradually weaning yourself off cigarettes when using them is just part of a routine. Ask yourself if there is enough variety in your meals so that you can turn to food for psychological contentment. Of course you will not want to allow food to replace cigarettes, which would result in overeating. You can learn to explore these issues and deal with them.

Smokers often use cigarettes when under stress. When Allison feels pressured, the first thing she does is reach for a cigarette. She says it helps her think. Is it because of that initial high that occurs when nicotine from the first few puffs hits the brain? You can learn how to think clearly without relying on cigarettes. Learning how to be in control of your life, and how to adopt a new perspective towards stressful situations, reduces the need to smoke. Changing your thinking and attitude towards the situation can allow you to reduce the number of times you need to turn to smoking or eating to relieve stress. You can learn how to relax naturally. If you opt for lifestyle change it will give you skills for a lifetime and allow you to get the full enjoyment out of life.

There are extra rewards for becoming a non-smoker. A recent study showed that by stopping smoking, even long-term smokers can reduce their risk of strokes to the same level as non-smokers within five years.[8] Within two years of stopping smoking, much of the tobacco-related risk of heart disease will also have disappeared.

HIGH CHOLESTEROL

Each year, according to the British Heart Foundation, 300,000 people in the U.K. die from heart disease. One of the major risk factors for heart disease is high blood cholesterol levels. As the artery openings become narrower, blood cannot pass through to carry oxygen and nutrients to the brain or heart (depending which artery is affected) and a stroke or heart attack will result.

Of the three major risk factors – smoking, high blood pressure and high cholesterol levels – the former two put the individual at a greater risk of heart disease. High cholesterol levels are a risk factor for heart disease in only a small percentage of cases. Since a risk factor is not a disease, is cholesterol becoming another word for paranoia?

According to Dr Corday, President of the American College of Cardiology and Clinical Professor of Medicine at the University of California Los Angeles, billions of dollars have been spent on studies investigating the link between cholesterol levels and heart disease. Billions more have been spent on campaigns encouraging people to reduce their cholesterol and now people are frightened to eat anything with cholesterol. Dr Corday states that the issue has made people neurotic about life and he expresses caution about the effects of restricting the cholesterol intake of children.

Cholesterol is especially important in the development of the nervous system during infancy and childhood. It is required to produce healthy cells in the body and brain, which is why it is particularly important for growing children. Feeding skimmed milk to children can be harmful for this reason.

There is no evidence that reduced cholesterol will extend life. On the other hand, adopting a healthier lifestyle can improve the quality of life. To help put the issue of cholesterol in perspective, several clients were plotted on the charts on the following pages to determine the overall risk of heart disease.

- Wayne had a high cholesterol level of 8.58 where 5.2 mmol/L or less is desirable. This fifty-one-year-old man was physically fit with good blood pressure (108/78) and he was a non-

FRAMINGHAM HEART STUDY – CHD RISK PREDICTION WORKSHEET

1. FIND POINTS FOR EACH RISK FACTOR.

Age (if female)

Age	Pts	Age	Pts	Age	Pts
30	-12	37	-2	46-47	5
31	-10	38	-1	48	6
32	-9	39	0	49-51	7
33	-7	40-41	1	52-53	8
34	-6	42	2	54-57	9
35	-5	43	3	58-61	10
36	-4	44-45	4	61-74	11

Age (if male)

Age	Pts	Age	Pts	Age	Pts
30	-2	42-43	6	59-60	14
31	-1	44	7	61-63	15
32-33	0	45-46	8	64-66	16
34	1	47-49	9	67-69	17
35-36	2	50-51	10	70-72	18
37	3	52-53	11	73-74	19
38-39	4	54-55	12		
40-41	5	56-58	13		

HDL Cholesterol – mmol/L

HDL-C	Pts	HDL-C	Pts	HDL-C	Pts
0.60-0.62	8	1.01-1.06	2	1.71-1.84	-4
0.65-0.67	7	1.09-1.16	1	1.87-2.02	-5
0.70-0.75	6	1.19-1.27	0	2.05-2.20	-6
0.78-0.83	5	1.29-1.40	-1	2.23-2.41	-7
0.85-0.90	4	1.42-1.53	-2	2.44-2.56	-8
0.93-0.98	3	1.55-1.68	-3		

Total Cholesterol – mmol/L

Total-C	Pts	Total-C	Pts
3.37-3.63	-4	5.67-6.19	2
3.65-3.96	-3	6.22-6.76	3
3.99-4.33	-2	6.79-7.38	4
4.35-4.72	-1	7.41-8.08	5
4.74-5.16	0	8.11-8.81	6
5.18-5.65	1		

Systolic Blood Pressure

SBP	Pts	SBP	Pts
95-97	-4	140-149	2
98-104	-3	150-159	3
105-112	-2	160-171	4
113-120	-1	172-184	5
121-129	0	185-190	6
130.139	1		

Other

Other	Pts
Cigarettes	4
Diabetic-male	3
Diabetic-female	6
ECG-LVH	9

0 pt for each NO

2. ADD UP POINTS FOR ALL RISK FACTORS

____ + ____ + ____ + ____ + ____ + ____ + ____ = ____

Age   Total-C   HDL-C   SBP   Smoker   Diabetes   ECG.LVH   Point total

Note: Minus points subtract from total

KEY: HDL-C = HDL Cholesterol; Total-C = Total Cholesterol; SBP = Systolic blood pressure (top number)

3. LOOK UP RISK CORRESPONDING TO POINT TOTAL

Pts	Probability 5 yr	10 yr	Pts	Probability 5 yr	10 yr	Pts	Probability 5 yr	10 yr	Pts	Probability 5 yr	10 yr
≤1	<1%	<2%	9	2%	5%	17	6%	13%	25	14%	27%
2	1%	2%	10	2%	6%	18	7%	15%	26	15%	29%
3	1%	2%	11	3%	7%	19	8%	16%	27	17%	31%
4	1%	2%	12	3%	7%	20	8%	18%	28	18%	33%
5	1%	3%	13	4%	8%	21	9%	19%	29	20%	35%
6	1%	3%	14	4%	9%	22	10%	21%	30	21%	37%
7	1%	4%	15	5%	11%	23	12%	23%	31	23%	39%
8	2%	4%	16	5%	12%	24	13%	25%	32	25%	42%

4. COMPARE TO AVERAGE 10 YEAR RISK

Age	Probability Women	Men	Age	Probability Women	Men	Age	Probability Women	Men
30-34	1%	3%	45-49	5%	10%	60-64	13%	21%
35-39	1%	5%	50-54	8%	14%	65-69	9%	30%
40-44	2%	6%	55-59	12%	16%	70-74	12%	24%

Kevin Anderson, Ph.D., Framingham Study; Dr W. B. Kannel, Boston University of Medicine[9]

5. NAME: _____   PT. TOTAL: _____   DATE: _____

smoker. He also had a healthy waist/hip ratio (more about this in Chapter 2).

- Robert, a large forty-six-year-old man, had an unhealthy waist/hip ratio, and a cholesterol level of 6.34. He did no exercise and smoked cigars. His blood pressure was 125/90 because his heart had to work harder due to his extra weight and poor fitness level. It takes an extra mile of blood vessels to nourish an extra pound of fat.

- Allen's only form of activity matched his Type A personality. His day was rush rush, got to get it done. His total cholesterol was 6.7, he had a healthy waist/hip ratio, and he was at a healthy weight for his height. His blood pressure was good at 106/70, but he smoked between ten and twenty cigarettes a day.

You will notice that Wayne, who was fitter than the other two, had the highest HDL (a cholesterol carrier that acts as your body's drain cleaner, different from the lazy cholesterol LDL) level of 1.47 which protected him against heart disease and lowered his overall risk. Allen's HDL value was 1.23 with Robert's trailing behind at 1.15.

	Age	Cholesterol	HDL	LDL	Triglycerides	BP	Smoker
Wayne	51	8.58	1.47	6.04	2.37	108/78	no
Robert	46	6.34	1.15	4.23	2.13	125/90	yes
Allen	49	6.70	1.23	4.60	1.92	106/70	yes

Following the above chart and working through Wayne's total points for all risk factors (based on the well-established Framingham Study referred to in more detail later in the book) it would look like this:

$$10 + (-2) + 6 + (-2) + 0 + 0 + 0 = 12$$

This means that even though the average risk for heart disease for a man Wayne's age within the next ten years is fourteen percent, the probability of his getting heart disease in that time frame is seven percent. His healthy blood pressure and high HDL value and the fact that he is a non-smoker make his high cholesterol level insignificant.

On the other hand, Robert's probability of getting heart disease within the next ten years is twelve percent, two points higher than the average of ten percent. Even though his cholesterol level is lower, his high blood pressure, minimal activity (which would result in a lower HDL value) as well as the fact that he is a smoker are higher risk factors for heart disease.

Allen is also a smoker, one of the major risk factors for heart disease. His risk of heart disease within the next ten years is about average at nine percent while the average for his age is ten percent.

These case studies show that it is better to focus on overall health rather than on one contributing factor, such as cholesterol. Yet too much misleading information on this subject has become a great source of concern for many people. You might like to consider the following facts:

- Blood cholesterol is a wax-like material produced in the liver and is used to make hormones, bile acids, and cell walls. HDL known as the 'good' cholesterol and LDL known as the 'bad' cholesterol are among the different types of cholesterol that are produced to make up the total cholesterol level in the body.

- Dietary cholesterol is found in all foods from animal sources, such as meat, eggs, and dairy products. However, *dietary cholesterol has a very small effect on blood cholesterol levels.*[10,11,12]

- 'I use 100 percent wholewheat bread with no cholesterol and no fat and add butter to it.' In this case the client's wise choice of bread is negated by the fact that he loads the bread with butter, the real culprit in raising cholesterol levels. Saturated fat is a key factor in raising blood cholesterol levels. Saturated fat can be defined as any fat that is hard at room temperature such as butter and lard. Other examples of hidden saturated fat could be processed meats such as sausages, luncheon meats, hot dogs, and dairy products such as cream, whole milk, cheese, and ice cream.

- Processing foods (e.g. peanut butter) can change a healthy kind of fat into one that will raise blood cholesterol levels. Convenience foods often contain palm and coconut oils, which are saturated fats that improve the shelf life of the product but also raise blood cholesterol levels. Peanut butter naturally contains the monounsaturated fat peanut oil which will not affect blood cholesterol levels. These types of fats are now being shown to possibly lower cholesterol levels.[13,14]

No one fat is better than another. A fat which is low in saturated fat, high in trans fatty acids, and contains hydrogenated vegetable oil, is the same as a fat that is high in saturated fat, contains no trans fatty acids and no hydrogenated vegetable oil. As a guide to your buying you could read the label! As soon as hydrogen is incorporated into the product to maintain shelf life (that is, keep it on the shelf without going rancid), it becomes hard at room temperature and is saturated. Therefore, hydrogenated peanut butter will raise your cholesterol level. *Note* Buy the natural peanut butter, stir it around, and keep it in the fridge. Some of my clients prefer to get rid of the fat on the surface altogether and add a little jam to it for moisture.

- Oils do not contain cholesterol. Cholesterol is made by the liver of an animal and since vegetable oils do not have livers, they cannot have any cholesterol! 'No cholesterol' could be featured on the label of all vegetable oils.

- Oat bran has some effect in lowering blood cholesterol levels. The exact mechanism by which the reduction occurs is uncertain. Recent studies suggest that incorporating oat bran or oatmeal into one diet reduces the overall saturated fat content of meals.[15]

- Polyunsaturated fats (corn oil, sunflower oil, and safflower oil) and monounsaturated fats (olive oil, peanut oil, canola) help to lower blood cholesterol levels. More recently, there has been a shift to the monounsaturated fats (olive, peanut, and canola or rapeseed oils) due to their effect on lowering LDL ('bad' cholesterol) without affecting the HDL ('good' cholesterol) that protects you from heart disease.[16]

But remember that it is not only a simple matter of switching the type of fat that you use, but of decreasing your total fat intake. Using a generous amount of olive oil to make pancakes makes this food higher in fat. Vary the types of fat you use from monounsaturated sources, but at the same time follow the suggestions presented to reduce the total fat in your cooking.

Eating a balance of more carbohydrates and less protein while including more sources of soluble fibre such as pulses (peas, beans, and lentils), fruits, and vegetables will help to lower cholesterol levels.

If you make a gradual change in your eating habits this will allow you to lower your blood cholesterol levels. Strict avoidance of certain foods only leads to cravings for those 'forbidden' items. In fact, the increased stress may offset any lowering of cholesterol levels that you are trying to effect by avoiding certain foods. You can reduce your cholesterol level naturally by learning how to acquire a taste for less fattening foods so that you can choose lower fat foods because you like them. Adding physical activity that you enjoy will help to increase the type of cholesterol (HDL) that will actually protect you from heart disease.

You can learn how to modify recipes during food preparation and baking to reduce fat content without removing the 'punch' in the meals. For example, gravy is great for adding flavour, moisture, and colour to your meal but is the fat really necessary?

You can learn how to read labels. If you know the real meaning of the word 'light' you can purchase products that are actually 'lighter' or lower in fat content rather than simply lighter in colour, taste, or texture. Gradually acquiring a taste for food with a lower fat content is the key to making a lower fat regime permanent.

Increasing aerobic activity increases HDL[17] which carries cholesterol out of the arteries to the liver where it is excreted from the body. This protects you against heart disease. On the other hand, lifestyle habits such as smoking can increase LDL (the lazy, sticky cholesterol carrier) which has the effect of plugging up your system by depositing cholesterol in the arteries. This adds to the risk of heart disease.

Your positive outlook on life in combination with a healthier lifestyle can improve your health status and lower your risk of heart disease.

PEOPLE WITH DIABETES

'It's supper time and I have to count out my exchanges to have the right balance according to my meal plan or diet sheet. I have to do this, not because I want to but because it's something that's controlling me. But some days I'm hungrier and some days I'm not. There's no flexibility.'

A person with diabetes maintains blood sugar control through the way they eat. Fortunately, the prescribed diabetic way of living is a healthy lifestyle. You can make the routine more 'normal' and flexible by making gradual lifestyle changes so you can begin to think like a non-dieter.

If you're on a diet, you may still want sweets but you try to say 'no' and you feel deprived. By learning to acquire a taste for less sugary foods, the power of choice rather than the diet sheet is the controlling mechanism. The blood sugar control will be achieved.

I have observed in the diabetic clinic over the past five years that those who adopt a more positive attitude are more relaxed with diabetes. They handle stress more positively and stabilise their blood sugar better than those who are worried and preoccupied with food and weight, portion control, and the 'magic' diet that they believe is the perfect way of eating. Lifestyle changes are less stressful and more positive than diets. They are for life!

Even the person with diabetes who is on insulin can benefit from a healthier way of thinking, can normalise eating and activity habits, and can work on skills to improve overall wellbeing. Consistency of carbohydrate intake and scheduled meals and snacks will be required to take account of the action of insulin, but empowering yourself to focus on health instead of diet details will make the process easier. You can make healthy living a choice that you desire!

Fluctuations in body weight are less healthy than if you stabilise at a higher weight.[18] Yo-yo dieting where weight is lost and then regained seems to be associated with more fat being distributed around the stomach area.[19] Increased risk of obesity-related diabetes has been associated with fat in the stomach area rather than fat in the hips and thighs.[20] As many as eighty percent of all people who have diabetes and are not on insulin are significantly overweight. By losing even a modest amount of weight, these patients may lower their insulin resistance to the point where the insulin their pancreases produce is sufficient to keep blood sugar levels down. A modest goal of a five or ten pound weight loss will often provide good results.[21,22]

Encouraging research indicates that physical training, even without weight loss, seems to increase the body's sensitivity to insulin, making the available insulin work harder. Aerobic exercise may improve the fit between insulin (key) and the cell receptor site (lock) allowing better control of blood sugar levels. Improvement can be noted in as little as one month after beginning a regular exercise programme. Within one year of doing this activity, aerobic exercise may even increase the number of receptor sites. Adjustment of diet also improves the insulin action within a matter of days even if body weight or body fat have decreased only slightly.[23]

Despite the benefits of an improved diet and exercise programme, estimates suggest that one third to one half of the people with diabetes have difficulty following these programmes for any length of time. Once blood sugar levels have been brought under control, old eating and exercise habits often return, along with the former lifestyle. Diet and exercise programmes treat diabetes but make little attempt to address the emotional response people have to food. Difficulties faced by people with diabetes are similar to those faced by other people who diet to try to lose weight:

- frequent feelings of hunger;
- feelings of restriction and deprivation due to elimination of some favourite foods;

- feelings of awkwardness at mealtimes because of eating differently from friends and family or because of having forced sudden changes in eating habits on the family;

- feelings of guilt when 'cheating', which inevitably occurs and often leads to going off the diet; and

- a feeling of total dependence on the diet sheet resulting in a total preoccupation with food.

Dieting for anyone is usually viewed as a stressful sacrifice. For people with diabetes, dieting is more stressful because of the consequences if they go off the diet. If people with diabetes add exercise that may be at too high a level resulting in pain, discomfort, and stiffness, they may give up and return to their former lifestyle. It's very important to find the balance that allows proper eating and appropriate activity for each individual.

For those people who have a genetic predisposition to diabetes, the disease will develop into Type II diabetes only if an abnormal weight gain occurs. People with diabetes who lead healthy lifestyles with regard to eating and exercise habits not only make their diabetes less severe and reduce the probability of complications, but also set an example of prevention for their children. For a person with diabetes, a minimal weight loss, especially early in the course of Type II diabetes, can cause diabetes to be reversed. A weight loss of five to ten kg (eleven to twenty-two pounds) is sufficient for diabetic control to be restored.[24] For diabetics on insulin, this approach can be used together wit the individual's diabetic meal plan. Check with your registered dietitian.

One of the ingredients of quality of life is to be in control of your life. The ability to direct the course of events in your life and being able to do what you want to do is challenged by having diabetes. This lifestyle approach to diabetes, leading to permanent adjustments in lifestyle through progressive gradual change, now offers the hope of less stressful and more lasting control of diabetes. It can give you the confidence to adopt a new lifestyle and to discard the perception that food controls you. *Special Note.* For those with diabetes, where regular products are mentioned in this book, low-sugar products need to be substituted. However, the key to long-term success is to acquire a taste for foods which are lower in sugar. Use the skills and techniques presented in this book to help you achieve this goal.

2

Resetting the Stage

Throw the scales away and focus on
rebuilding your health

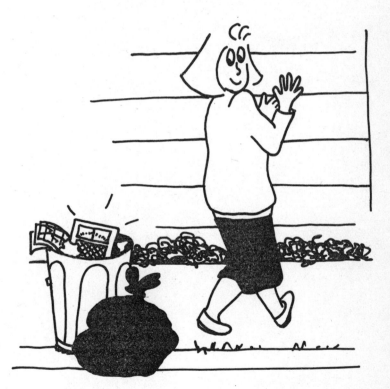

THE ALMIGHTY SCALE

For many of us, the scale rules our lives. It has the power to dictate what we eat, how we feel, and how we act. We weigh in and according to the needle indicator we feel happy or depressed. Eighty percent of the women in Canada believe they are overweight, yet the Canada Fitness Survey indicates that only twenty percent of women over twenty years of age experience a health risk due to excess body weight. This same survey shows that thirty-three percent of Canadian men have a health risk because of excess body weight. Men are at a higher health risk because of obesity, yet women are more preoccupied with food and the number on the scale.

In fact, many women allow the number on the scale to put their life on hold until they reach their ideal weight. This obsession with weight prevents them from getting on with their lives. They rationalise: 'I'll be happy only when I've lost ten pounds. I'll start exercising once I've lost the weight. I don't look good in a track suit now.' Unfortunately this kind of weight loss is usually temporary. Your moments of happiness are gone when you gain back what you lost and the cycle begins again. Your weight problem is not solved and your self-esteem gets lower and lower.

When did this preoccupation with weight begin? Probably in the late 50s when the new Metropolitan height/weight tables came out followed by Twiggy's shape in the 60s. Women discovered that according to the tables they were ten pounds overweight and the image that was projected in the media reinforced an ever slimmer figure.

Dieting began as women tried to obtain the ideal figure. The intense pressure that society's cultural values place on women to conform to specific body shapes creates an obsession with external appearance at the expense of basic body needs. Focusing on the scales ties your self-worth and self-esteem to an external artificial cue and doesn't allow you to discover yourself and pay attention to your body's needs. It prevents inner growth.

Because you admire society's ideal shape and want to lose weight to obtain it, you are temporarily motivated to pursue a diet and lose the pounds. But you haven't dealt with why you overate in the first place, so when you stop the diet and the weight returns you are devastated. Focusing on a lifestyle change that will deal with the basics of your problem is the only way that you can prevent this up-and-down cycle and the depression that accompanies it. In order to use lifestyle change as a measure of success, let go of the control the scale has over you.

The Yo-Yo Syndrome

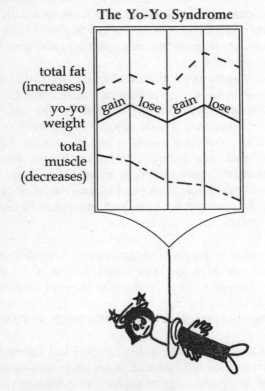

total fat
(increases)

yo-yo
weight

total
muscle
(decreases)

gain lose gain lose

Deanna, aged eighteen, came to see me for weight loss. She had been in a weight-loss programme and her mother was attending one of the popular weight-loss programmes and was constantly on and off a diet. Deanna and her mother both attended the first session with me. Her mother remarked that I was trying to deprogramme them from the diet mentality. That was true. No diets and no scales were involved in what I had to say.

A few months later, Deanna said that her clothes felt looser and she and her mother were curious to know if she had lost weight. Deanna was down two sizes, yet she had lost only five pounds. She had a noticeable improvement in her waist/hip ratio (from .80 to .73) which means that she was healthier. Her menstrual period resumed, and she was no longer cranky or grouchy. She was eating only until she was satisfied, not stuffed. She was more energetic.

It was obvious that the scales had not told the true story. The composition of weight for each pound lost during the first three days on a 1500 calorie weight-loss diet is seventy percent water, five percent protein, and twenty-five percent fat.[1] Over the long term, without exercise, only fifty percent of the weight is lost as fat, the rest is muscle tissue and water. The big weight loss the scales indicate is water loss. This deceives the dieter into believing that progress is being made – until the weight comes back.

Since muscles burn more calories at rest, they are more metabolically active than fat is. The trouble is that when we lose weight, we lose some of that tissue, and when it is gained back, we gain back more fat (see graph p42). The result may be less on the scale, but we have traded valuable muscle tissue for fat.[2]

Muscle weighs more than fat since it needs to be stored with water. So if we gain more muscle, we may not lose as much on the scale or may actually gain some weight. Exercise preserves muscle mass. As the saying goes, 'If you don't use it, you'll lose it.' What counts is not how much you weigh, but how much of that weight is fat.

Women are often concerned about large hips. Yet nature intended it that way. This extra fat around the hip area is to protect women in childbearing so they will have enough energy

stores to call on. Fat around the stomach area is a higher health
risk, and is lost more easily than fat situated lower on the body.

Take a moment to determine your present waist/hip ratio, a
measure that will be used to check your indicator of health risk.
You can throw out the scales. From now on use the waist/hip
ratio to replace it.

With a tape measure, measure your girth at the waist, at your
navel, and around your hips at their widest point. Be consistent
each time you measure. Be careful not to measure more
frequently than once every few months. Otherwise, the obsession wit the scale may be inappropriately replaced by a new
crutch, the waist/hip ratio. The purpose of this measurement is
simply to provide a periodic indication for those individuals
who wear loose-fitting clothes and are therefore unable to
measure change by the way their clothes fit. Normal values
are 0.8 for woman and 1.0 for men.

Measure of Health (Annual Health Log)

	Begin	3 Months	6 Months	9 Months	12 Months
Waist					
Hip					
Waist/Hip Ratio					

** The risk increases sharply when the ratio of waist to hip circumference
exceeds 1.0 in men and 0.8 in women.*

This example is for a full-figured woman and demonstrates
that a larger body size does not necessarily determine one's
health status.

Female   waist 40 inches
             hips 50 inches
             waist/hip ratio   40/50 = 0.8

This means that this woman's waist is eighty percent of her hip
measurement, or putting it another way her waist is twenty

percent less than her hips. This ratio gives her a slight curvature. Since fat around the waist determines the risk of heart disease, high blood pressure, and diabetes, this woman whose fat is more concentrated around her hips is at a lower risk for these diseases.

Male   waist 50 inches
       hips 40 inches
       waist/hip ratio   50/40 = 1.25

This signifies that this man has a pot belly. The weight concentrated around the waist represents a higher health risk. He is more apple-shaped, in contrast to the woman who is more pear-shaped.

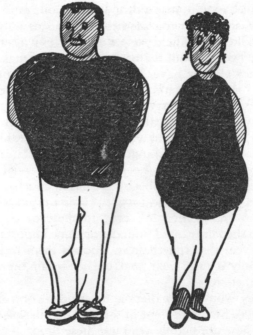

Don't despair! Fat comes off easiest from the waist, the area which lowers your waist/hip ratio and improves your health status.[3] Now plot your own waist/hip ratio on the chart above, and note your progress on a quarterly basis by retaking measurements.

REALITIES OF DIETING

Most people go on diets to lose weight quickly. If quick weight loss does not occur they become bored and are not motivated to stay on the diet. According to some scientists, quick weight loss is pointless because these individuals are being set up to gain that weight back very quickly.

Individuals focusing on achieving quick weight loss usually do well for a few months. Then, with a loss of interest or as they reach a plateau, weight gain inevitably occurs. These individuals are not in tune with their body's needs, which is why they put weight on in the first place. The half pound per week weight loss recommended to minimise a drop in metabolic rate[4] is exceeded on quick weight-loss programmes which focus only on weight and not on lifestyle. These people need to look a certain way in order to feel good about themselves, instead of making the best of what they already have. Rather than focusing on one event and living for the moment, they could take a broader focus and enjoy the process of lifestyle change.

Losing weight quickly causes the weight to return three times as quickly. Dr Wayne Callaway, Associate Clinical Professor of Medicine at George Washington University, stated that, with rare exceptions, none of the popular commercially available programmes for treating obesity are based on current scientific knowledge. They could no longer promise rapid weight loss if they were.[5] Yet women fall prey to these quick weight-loss schemes to shed unwanted pounds for some important occasion or social event that they believe requires them to be slimmer. Some actually achieve their goal, only to regain the weight once the crash diet stops.[6].

Laxatives won't help dieting or weight control. Approximately five to fifteen percent of the U.S. population are laxative abusers. These are people who use these drugs at least weekly for several months. They include not only many elderly patients but also individuals with eating disorders and others who are preoccupied with weight. However, studies have shown that a maximum of only twelve percent of calories are unabsorbed as a result of laxatives.[7] Laxatives are not a quick fix.

If you take regular exercise and enjoy healthy eating by

putting food in its proper perspective, your body will do the work for you to get you to the size which is right for you. According to Dr David Williamson, an epidemiologist at the Centre for Disease Control in Atlanta, it may be better for a woman in the long term to maintain a given weight, and focus efforts on counselling to accept herself and how she views herself at her current weight, unless the weight is actually causing some medical problems.

When someone has heart disease, diabetes, high blood pressure, or any ailment, they are told to lose weight. Yet in a study of a community with a high incidence of overweight but in which obesity was socially acceptable, levels of heart disease and diabetes were found to be below the average for slender Americans.[8] It is losing the weight and gaining it back, known as 'weight cycling', that makes one more susceptible to disease.[9] The obsession to be thin causes more people to be on a diet than off a diet at any given time.[10]

It is not how much you weigh that counts, but rather where the fat is distributed.[11] Stabilising at a higher weight is actually healthier than yo-yo dieting.[12] This shift of weight down and then up results in a higher percentage of upper body fat distribution, in other words, more fat in the stomach area.[13] This tendency to carry fat in the upper body is associated with a higher risk of diabetes, high blood pressure, and heart disease.[14,15] Rather than concentrating on weight loss, focus on health and wellness.

Enjoying the process of self-discovery associated with lifestyle changes lasts a lifetime. During the YCCD programme, the involvement and enthusiasm of participants are high, and this results in steady progress in lifestyle changes. However, in Jill's case, her progress led her to believe that she could tackle the internalisation of lifestyle changes on her own. Her success was short-lived. She was intimidated by projected media images of slim, svelte, 'perfect' bodies and this destroyed her progress towards her personal goal. She joined yet another diet programme. Success was once again measured by the number on the scale. She was creating a stressful situation for herself, and the physical and psychological shortcomings of dieting resulted in eventual weight gain. It is interesting how many times we have to reach the wall in order to realise that **diets do not work**.

Another example may also be convincing. Kerry participated in the YCCD programme in its developmental stages when it was still focused on diet, exercise, and behaviour modification. Kerry lost weight and, in fact, a year later when I saw here she was even slimmer, almost too slim. I spoke to her about how the programme had evolved to a non-dieting approach to healthy living. She was not very receptive because she was doing well on her diet. Her focus was to eat and exercise in the right way for weight loss. Finally, however, the constant deprivation caused cravings for food that resulted in binging on chips, cheesecake, and all those 'forbidden' foods that were now unbearably enticing.

Once Kerry began to regain weight she was interested in hearing the YCCD message. Her body was going through a normal reaction as she was rebelling against dieting. Binging does not occur without periods of restriction (dieting). Kerry realised that it was only by changing her thinking that she would be able to prevent more weight gain.

It is true that stressful situations may cause you to go off the diet; but lifestyle changes help you to deal with stressful situations more positively, allowing you to learn from your mistakes and accept life's hills and valleys as challenges. Diets which cause body stress are difficult to maintain when stressful situations occur. Since life is filled with everyday stresses, you need the tools to handle stress positively.

As you have seen, diets and scales are not the answer to weight problems. I hope by now you have been convinced to put the scales in the cupboard. If you are unable to let go, your preoccupation with your weight can prevent you from focusing on lifestyle changes. If you think you can do both, think again. By worrying about your weight and feeling unhappy about the way you look, this unhealthy attitude will lead to an energy drain and you will lose your motivation to correct your lifestyle and lose weight permanently.

This book focuses on lifestyle skills that you can use for a lifetime. The results will be increased self-esteem, improvement in overall health, and increased energy. You will accept yourself the way you are and use newly learned skills to focus on your strengths and work on your weaknesses.

Accepting yourself the way you are is one of the most difficult skills to master. Most of us have been conditioned to believe that we should aim for size 10 or even size 6. However, only ten percent of the population can naturally fall into this category.

Instead of having to be thin to feel good about yourself, reverse the process. You have to accept yourself and feel good about yourself first in order to want to nurture yourself and take care of your body and mind. Accepting yourself as you are does not mean that you are absolutely okay and you will do nothing to improve yourself. Rather, it implies that you have the energy to feel good about yourself, and because you do care about yourself, you want to do what is best for your body and mind so that you can be the best that you can be!

Gradually this mindset will become part of your daily life and will enable you to start each day on a positive note. This is a very important step. Give yourself time to gain confidence. It will happen if you believe it can and take the steps to increase the chances.

Being unhappy with the way you look provides only temporary external motivation which usually results in a diet and eventually weight gain. When you focus on the positive, you will move forward on your road to better health. You will gradually learn to tune into your body, and when you understand your body you will learn to fuel your body according to its needs. Accepting yourself allows you to understand these needs and listen to your body more attentively. Your body will naturally adjust to what it is meant to be. This will help you to stabilise your weight. No more up-and-down weight and no more diets!

Let's go one step further. In order to focus on lifestyle changes you need to accept that diets don't work. Remember that a lot of the weight lost when dieting is due to dehydration (water loss). Even some popular 'balanced' diets are relatively low on carbohydrates. So when you start depleting or getting rid of your carbohydrate stores (glycogen), out goes the water too. No wonder you are always running to the toilet, since every pound of glycogen is stored with three to four pounds of water. Restricting carbohydrate foods such as potatoes, bread, cereals, pasta, and rice leads to an energy drain along with your dehydrated state. No wonder you get irritable!

Practise saying these phrases to yourself first thing in the morning and last thing at night

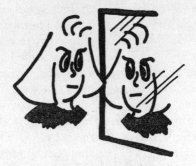

'I like myself.'

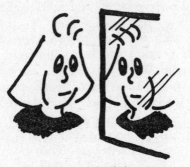

'I am a worthwhile person!'

'I am going to have a great day!'

Caught in a vicious diet circle?

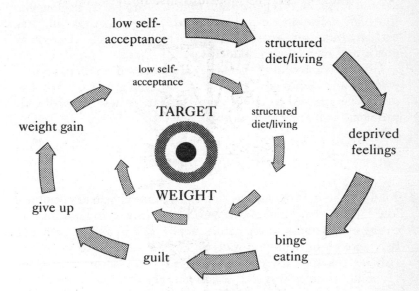

low self-acceptance → structured diet/living

low self-acceptance

TARGET

structured diet/living

weight gain

WEIGHT

deprived feelings

give up

binge eating

guilt

THE YCCD HEALTHY LIVING CYCLE!

A positive, energetic approach that improves your mental and physical health. It just keeps getting better as you repeat the cycle!

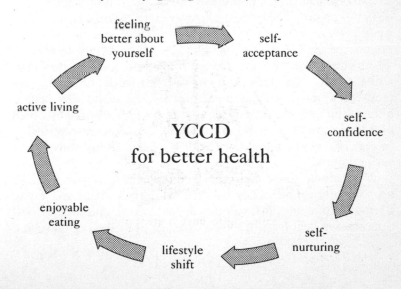

feeling better about yourself → self-acceptance

active living

YCCD for better health

self-confidence

enjoyable eating

self-nurturing

lifestyle shift

The diet fad of the 80s was to reduce carbohydrates, resulting in energy drain. The calorie-obsessed, protein-is-in, starches-are-out habits of this generation of adults are partly responsible for high rates of cancer and heart disease. After all, less carbohydrate automatically implies higher protein content at meals and that is more hidden fat.

Now a new round of diets is evolving based on an obsession with fat and cholesterol. Instead of counting grams of carbohydrate, we are told to count grams of fat. A new set of health problems will emerge from this.

DIETS AREN'T THE ANSWER[16]

John had an iron deficiency. For eight months he had been on a low-fat diet that he considered to be healthy. After all, he was eating more fruits and vegetables, very little fat, and chicken and fish were his only protein sources. He was not eating any foods rich in iron such as red meat and any iron he ingested from vegetable sources was not effectively absorbed because of his consumption of coffee with his meals (see Chapter 11 for more detail). John ate very little bread and cereals, which are rich in vitamin B, and his low-fat diet probably impaired the absorption of some fat-soluble vitamins such as A, D, E, and K.

His reason for going on the diet in the first place was to lose weight. He lost fifteen pounds in the first two months. Then he began to go on and off the diet. After eight months his constant weight fluctuation had provided a weight loss of only five pounds below his starting weight. John loved fatty foods and whenever he went off the diet he binged on some of these fat-laden foods. His unhealthy attitude towards food and his temporary drastic change in eating because of his diet caused a starve/binge cycle and consequent up-and-down weight which provided a greater risk of heart disease. It took some convincing to make him realise that he was doing harm to his body by his eating habits.

What about those diets that reduce calorie intake and are nutritionally sound? They don't work either. After all, if you normally consume 2000 calories a day, you would have a hard time staying healthy on 1200 calories, or even staying on such a diet for a long time without becoming physically incapaci-tated.[17] Did you ever notice that after a few weeks of losing weight you reach a plateau and you don't lose weight anymore. Think about why this happens and it will help you to under-stand why diets don't work.

The plateau occurs because of a drop in metabolic rate, the number of calories that the body burns at rest in order for your heart to pump, your blood to flow, and your lungs to work. **When you begin a calorie-reduced diet your metabolic rate drops fifteen to thirty percent within twenty-four to forty-eight hours.**[18] When you diet, your body slows itself down and packs on a bit more fat so that it has something to call on when you put it in a starvation situation again. It is your body's natural reaction in order to defend you from the sudden drop in calories that you are experiencing.

Eventually, when you deprive yourself of food to reduce your calorie intake, especially if it's the kind of food you like or the quantities you are used to consuming, you won't be able to maintain the diet. For some people, even the thought of going on a diet conjures up a desire for those forbidden foods, and the cravings are too strong to resist.

You Didn't Fail. Diets Failed You.
It's easy to cheat but it's always accompanied by feelings of guilt. In this way we are not extracting the full enjoyment from food and need more food to derive psychological satisfaction. If diets worked, there would not be a new one on the market all the time. People would not have to go back to the same programme over and over again for the rest of their lives.

Unfortunately, during the loss-and-gain cycle of a weight-loss diet you lose the same twenty pounds over and over again. Each time the weight comes back it's more difficult to lose and easier to put back on. In fact, diets make you fatter. What about the traditional safe weight loss of one to two pounds per week, you ask? This may be safe but even these diets cause dieters to experience a drop in their metabolic rate. Most dieters (ninety-five percent) who lose weight regain the weight within a five-year period and many gain back even more than they lost.[19] It's nature's way of protecting you for the next onslaught of deprivation.[20]

Some film stars, for example Delta Burke from *Designing Women*, are promoting new ways of thinking about their own bodies and dieting. In an interview with *National Enquirer* she states 'You can make the most of your shape with good nutrition and exercise for fitness, but you can't make yourself tall and willowy if your body type is squat and muscular.' She goes on to say that the only answer is to accept the body type you were born with, and learn to feel comfortable in your own skin. People weren't meant to be like peas in a pod, and wouldn't it be boring if we were all the same?

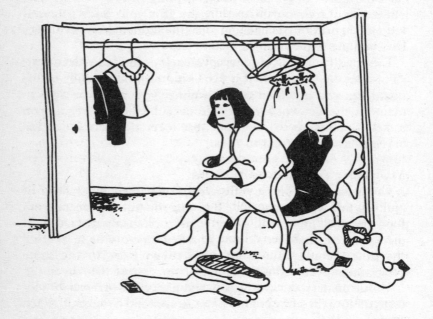

Take the first step. Start right now by accepting your body and stop separating your wardrobe into thin clothes and fat clothes. Stop concentrating on the hope of being thin again and make the most of what you have right now. You're you and proud of it. The next time you go shopping treat yourself to a new outfit that looks good on you right now. Learn to accent your best features. It's amazing the lift in energy this will give you, and it will help to channel that energy so you will take care of the rest of your body. Accepting the way you are is a lot easier if you help it along with something nice that will make you feel better immediately. Stop punishing yourself and start pampering yourself. You are worth the effort!

Calories don't count. It is not how much you eat, but the type of food you eat that counts.[21] It takes about four times the calories to convert carbohydrates into fat than it does to convert the fat you eat into fat tissue.[22] Switching to eating more carbohydrates without guilt allows you to shift the type of calories you eat without significantly changing the total quantity of calories. This minimises the drop in metabolic rate.[23]

This may be a difficult concept to grasp since it is the direct reverse of what many dieters are used to hearing. 'How can I expect to eat properly and in a healthy manner and expect to lose weight?' you ask. My reply is a question also. 'Do you have to subject your body to some type of torture, denial, and restriction in order to feel that you are accomplishing something? When you exercise do you expect to feel pain in order that you have had a good workout?'

The secret is to enjoy food to the full while you are eating. If you do not allow yourself the enjoyment of tasting and savouring the food without guilt, you will be hungry later on. You will need more food to satisfy you psychologically since you were not focusing on your food while you were eating. Remember, eating bread (carbohydrates) does not mean eating the whole loaf. You need to understand your body's needs and change your thinking about food so you can take charge of your eating.

An increase in calories, especially carbohydrates, is necessary to increase your metabolic rate. Most diets are low in carbohydrates to initiate immediate weight loss. It is the depletion of carbohydrate stores which results in water loss that makes the scales register weight loss. Eventually the incomplete breakdown of fat produces ketone bodies. This is a very unhealthy way of losing weight.[24] It is also very temporary, since rehydration occurs once carbohydrates are eaten again. An example of this would be losing weight to get into that special dress for the wedding only to regain the weight (rehydrate) by eating some cake at the wedding. 'I only have to look at cake and I gain weight,' you say. In order to minimise the feelings of deprivation and to make healthy eating a lifestyle change it must be done gradually so there is no shock to your body.

HOW DIETS RULE YOU

- Diets decrease metabolism, slowing your motor down to a halt as you eat less and less to prevent weight gain.

- Diets foster poor eating habits which lead to periods of starving and binging.

- Diets decrease your self-esteem because the weight comes back and you feel that you are a failure. In this way your self-worth is tied to the number on the scales.

HEALTHY LIFESTYLE PUTS YOU IN CHARGE

- Stop dieting and get your metabolism moving again. Food of the proper types will get your system revved up again.

- Eating regularly and not starving yourself prevents overeating. If you know you can have it, the desire for it is less.

- Don't equate self-worth with the number on the scales. Focus on health rather than weight. Throw the scales into the dustbin and take control of your health.

DOES SLIMNESS EQUAL HEALTH?

According to Ellen Parham,[25] a new set of goals and benefits for health can be defined.

- Relieve a health problem.

- Increase your self-esteem.

- Achieve a sense of control over your eating.
- Improve nutritive adequacy.
- Increase fitness and flexibility through exercise.
- Develop a lifestyle that will reduce the risk of obesity for yourself and others.

Think about these alternatives. They can help you to be successful.

Many slim people compromise their health to retain their ideal figure. How do they do it?

- Are they starving and binging?
- Are they more preoccupied with food and weight?
- Is their life focused around food?
- Are they over-exercising?
- Are they happy with their lives and their bodies?
- Are they using cigarettes to control their weight?
- Do they get more colds; are they sick more frequently?

Dieting exacts its price. Protein breakdown results in breakdown of the immune system which makes you more susceptible to disease. The physical and mental stress of dieting weakens the immune system. According to scientific studies, deficiencies of protein and some amino acids, the building blocks of protein, as well as vitamins A, E, B6, folate, zinc, iron, and copper are associated with reduced functioning of the immune system which wards off disease.[26] Some research indicates that even mild upsets causing swings in daily mood can disturb the immune system. Since the immune system is the central link that controls disorders such as heart disease and cancer, upsetting this balance is not good for the body.

Many film stars and models undereat and overexercise to maintain their figures. Since their careers are built on 'ideal' shapes they can't afford to lose them. Cher exercises two hours or more every day. She eats very little, but if she overeats or will be appearing in public, she increases her exercise up to four hours a day. Kenny Rogers, who has tried every diet without success, had fat surgically removed from his stomach and chin. Dolly Parton, Jane Fonda, and Karen Carpenter all suffered from anorexia nervosa. In fact, Karen Carpenter died in 1983 from a heart attack brought on by complications as a result of this eating disorder.

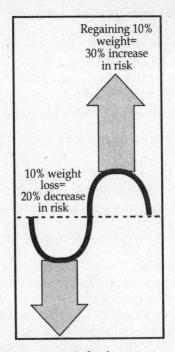

Relationship between weight loss/gain and the risk of heart disease

Fluctuation in body weight due to yo-yo dieting is more harmful to your health than stabilising at a higher weight.[27] It causes an increased risk of heart disease, gallstones, and high blood pressure. In the Framingham Heart Study, which monitored more than 5,000 people for forty years, the following was reported:

- people who lost ten percent of their body weight had a twenty percent reduction in risk of heart disease.

- people who gained back ten percent of their body weight increased risk of heart disease to thirty percent.[28]

In other words, stabilising at a higher weight is healthier (i.e. twenty percent increase in heart disease) than losing and then regaining weight (i.e. thirty percent increase in heart disease).[29] Genetically, if both parents are large, children have an eighty percent chance of being large. If one parent is large, children have a fifty percent chance of being large.

We are not all meant to be thin even though slim females and lean muscular models are paraded before us as ideals. In reality, there is no perfectly shaped person without the help of plastic surgery.

Three Main Body Types
Endomorph heavy build, rounded on all sides, shoulders often narrower than hips, higher percentages of body fat, often carried on the hips, waist, thighs, and buttocks; stocky individuals with round body features, prominent abdominal viscera, large trunk and thighs, and tapering extremities.

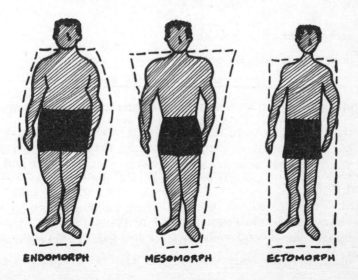

ENDOMORPH   MESOMORPH   ECTOMORPH

Mesomorph broad shoulders and some narrowness in the rib cage, waist, and hips; weight concentrated in the upper body, giving them extra power and strength, more muscular than other body types, relatively predominantly bony and muscular framework, strong physique.

Ectomorph tall, slim body, small-framed with narrow shoulders, hips often narrower than shoulders, low levels of body fat, low muscularity.

If you understand and appreciate your body you will be able to work with it, not against it. You cannot become another type. No matter how you starve yourself, your basic body shape will remain.

This programme will allow you to work with your body and develop your full potential. It will show you a new way of thinking about yourself. Acknowledging two basic premises is crucial to allowing you to move forward in this programme. You must accept yourself as you are and develop your potential, and you must be convinced that diets don't work. Now you can forget past failures and move into a positive future. You're doing very well. Now, check the following chart to make sure you are ready to proceed. In order to make lifestyle changes you need to:

- accept yourself as you are;
- believe that diets do not work;
- give up past failures and move on to the present;
- give up judging your self-worth by the number on the scale;
- trust your ability to let go and relax and allow changes to happen naturally rather than forcing them; by letting go, you are better able to experience who you really are and to give yourself permission to develop and become your true self;
- get more in touch with yourself to recognise your internal hunger signals and your physical and psychological needs;
- listen to your body with regard to food intake, physical

activity and its intensity and benefits, as well as the need to schedule special time for yourself; and

- begin to observe how dieters and non-dieters handle situations differently, especially with regard to food.

Discuss our philosophy with your friends and family so they do not sabotage your efforts. Otherwise if they think you are on a diet and catch you eating a piece of cake or some biscuits they may try to make you feel guilty. This can lead you to eat more, since you are being robbed of the satisfaction from the piece that you ate. This can once again lead to 'secret eating' which puts you right back into the diet mentality.

LIFE EXPECTANCY VERSUS HEALTH EXPECTANCY

My dentist told me that he heard a renowned speaker say that dieting to achieve ideal body weight improves how long you live by only a few years. So what's the point of giving up those foods you like. 'I want to live and I want to die happy,' was my dentist's conclusion.

What he said is true up to a point. Achieving ideal weight for large people, as a group, would gain an average of only 0.7 to 1.7 years for men, and 0.5 to 1.1 years for women. Further evidence suggests that lowering the risk factors of high blood pressure and high serum cholesterol to recommended levels would add 1.1 to 5.3 and 0.5 to 4.2 years, respectively, for men; 0.9 to 5.7 and 0.4 to 6.3 for women. Further evidence shows that male smokers, as a whole, would gain 2.3 years from stopping smoking; female smokers 2.8 years.[30] These projected gains from weight loss are minimal. So if this is the case, why are we as a society focusing on weight to begin with? Is doing the bare minimum in order to live longer the answer? What about quality of life?

Some studies indicate that twenty million Americans will be over the age of eighty-five by the year 2000. This may indicate their life expectancy but what about their health expectancy, which is a measure of their quality of life? Health expectancy indicates how long you are likely to be healthy and active, rather than how many years you may live. Let's compare the health expectancies of two individuals who live to the same age. Person A smokes, is overweight, and has high cholesterol. This person develops heart disease at the age of fifty, emphysema by the age of sixty, and lung cancer at seventy-five. The later years are filled with pain, mental depression, financial problems, and emotional isolation. Person B does not smoke or have high cholesterol and is a healthy weight. Because of hereditary factors, Person B develops heart disease at the age of seventy-five. The later years for Person B are vital and fulfilling up until death. When preparing for the later years, investing in your health now may be as important as investing your money for retirement.

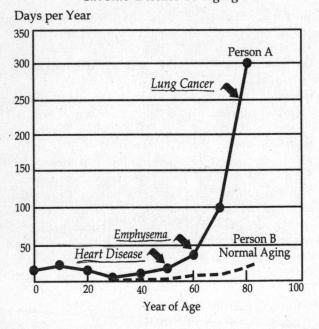

Annual Restricted Activity Days
Chronic Disease vs Aging

(from The National Centre for Health Statistics)

Giving up the foods you like is not where we're heading. My dentist was partly correct when he said 'I eat what I want and enjoy it.' We want you to do this. The difference is to retrain your taste buds so that you acquire a taste for healthier foods. The roller coaster effect of cutting out all fats even though you may enjoy these foods is not the answer. Such a drastic denial only leads to feelings of deprivation and cannot be maintained. Take it slowly and gradually for lasting effects.

Low-fat foods that my dentist thinks will be the answer to the fat problem won't help him to acquire a taste for healthier foods. Just as sugar substitutes don't make a person lose the taste for sweets. My dentist's theory is that sugar substitutes cause us to indulge in more fats. Is it that the sugar substitutes are not satisfying enough? The incidence of obesity has not decreased. Since low-fat products will have few calories we probably will eat more of them. But are we solving the basic problem or are we fooling ourselves into believing that we are actually improving our health?

It's human nature to want instant gratification, instant success. Why bother trying to modify eating habits when a fat substitute will do the trick? The answer is healthy living. It's the long term that's important.

Being healthy is the key. The proper weight for each individual, which is called the setpoint, should be the focus for health. Listen to your body. It will guide you to the right weight for you. Accept yourself as you are. **You don't have to try to remake yourself according to someone else's fantasy.**

Having an open mind, learning to fine-tune our present lifestyle and making small gradual changes will build the foundation for a healthier way of living.

ACTION POINTS

● Throw away the scales.

● Identify and write ways to shift your focus to good health and away from weight loss. Stop dieting.

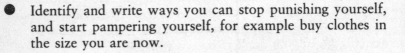

● Identify and write ways you can stop punishing yourself, and start pampering yourself, for example buy clothes in the size you are now.

● Say affirmations regularly:

'I like myself.'

'I am a worthwhile person.'

'I am going to have a great day.'

● Use waist–hip ratio as a health indicator instead of focusing on weight. Be careful not to get hooked into replacing the crutch and obsession of the scales with a new number. Once you tune into how your body feels, numbers won't even be necessary.

● Re-read the check list on p60 to help get yourself into a positive frame of mind to move forward.

3

Physical Activity for Pleasure

Exercise regularly at your own level with an
activity you enjoy

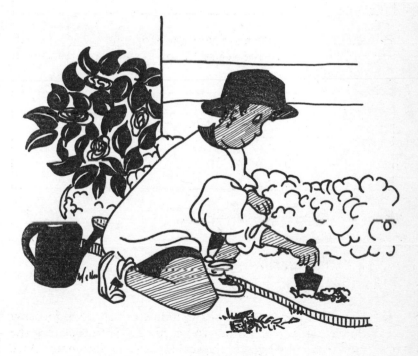

The YCCD principle is focused on lifestyle change that you allow to happen naturally. In order to make your activity level a lifestyle change, it must be increased gradually. It's important to find an activity that you truly enjoy so you feel you are doing it for yourself, not because you have to do it. For this to happen, it is necessary to understand the principles of fitness in relation to this programme.

Part of the balance sought in lifestyle change is that daily physical activity is to be enjoyed. This refers to the normal day-to-day movement of a moderately active person going about the business of living. Called 'active living', it involves such activities as getting up, getting dressed, working, lifting things, putting them down, walking around, doing housework, going out in the evening, etc. Active living burns twenty-five percent of your total calories if you are moderately active. However, most people are not moderately active and when they do not reach their calorie burning potential they retain the calories and accumulate fat.

In the past, exercise was viewed as a form of punishment rather than reward. Push-ups or running around the block were activities forced on you if you were bad. Aerobics was also hard work. Each evening you went to the fitness club, and put up with the hour of pain. No gain without pain, you thought. You continued out of perseverance or after a few months gave it up, feeling that exercise was not for you.

My own experience of attending regular aerobic classes was that I felt exhausted. I was often dizzy and in pain, but I thought this was a normal reaction and I wanted to be in shape. But when the soreness and stiffness persisted I decided to give up aerobics. A few years later, with new knowledge and a new attitude, I tackled other types of physical activity. It's now three years later and I enjoy exercising, mainly walking and cycling. Now I teach aerobic classes at a lower intensity that emphasises enjoyment.

We encourage back-to-basics active living which is a self-paced, integrated activity, working out in more natural surroundings, such as your garden, a playground, or skating rink. It involves natural movements used in everyday living. Sustained, strenuous exercise is now thought to be unnecessary according to some fitness experts. You need only take the equivalent of a few brisk walks weekly to increase your likelihood of living a long and healthy life.

Living actively rewards you twice: immediately, in the pleasure of doing the activity, and over time, through improved health, wellbeing, and quality of life. Moving the way you like to move is good for you. It's the moving that counts.

Active living refers to enjoying physical activity and learning how to integrate it into your daily life. This indicates that longevity is enhanced through any kind of activity and that people can be fit by doing ordinary, useful activities whether it is decorating your home, cleaning your bathroom, or working in the garden.

You can pursue this active living at work as well. Take the stairs instead of the lift; put a pair of walking shoes in your car and take a walk if you're early for an appointment; walk around the block after lunch before returning to work; park your car a distance away from your workplace so that you can enjoy a short walk before the day's activities. These lifestyle moves do not even take extra time; rather they give you time. These changes get you moving and keep you moving. They lead to more energy and a healthier and longer lifespan.

Dependence on fitness classes or other structured physical activity to get fit does not work in the long term. It's the same kind of dependence that people place on a diet club. They follow the diet as long as they are involved in a group situation to reinforce and encourage them. They go off the diet as soon as they stop attending classes. When the reason for doing exercise is weight loss and not fun, people find excuses not to go to classes. The focus of exercise should be to encourage self-awareness so that active living becomes the answer to exercise needs.

Active living is an entirely different way of viewing activity. It promotes enjoyment of life and the awareness of what is going on around you. The main focus is to make choices for yourself, based on what you want and enjoy. Then you will find new excitement in activity and it will become a pleasurable part of your life. If you listen to your body and tune into your body's needs you will know what intensity of activity you should follow.

MYTHS OF EXERCISING

Myth 1: No pain, no gain
Painful, intense exercising will not lead to lifestyle change. Continued discomfort will discourage you from continuing the exercise. In fact, painful exercise can damage your body. New fitness information emphasises 'train but not strain'. The old pain-for-gain thinking destroys the sense of fun and enjoyment and does not fit into your new active lifestyle.

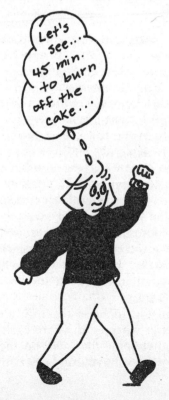

Forget the old way: 'I went for a walk to the cake shop where I can have one as my reward,' or 'I ate a piece of cake, so I'll have to walk it off.' Activity is for pleasure, which in itself is the reward. The old 'calories taken in versus calories used up' attitude traps you in the diet mentality of counting calories. You ask yourself whether exercise is really worth the effort. You walk a half hour to the cake shop so that you have used up enough calories to reward yourself with a small doughnut. The sense of discouragement that develops further depletes your energy and results in a poor attitude towards exercise.

		Exercise needed to use up calories		
Calories Taken In		*WALKING*	*BICYCLING*	*RUNNING*
Average cake	150 calories	29 min.	18 min.	8 min.
1 slice cheesecake	260 calories	50 min.	32 min.	13 min.
1/6 of fruit tart	410 calories	79 min.	50 min.	21 min.

Normal glycogen (carbohydrate) stores provide fuel for about two hours of moderate-intensity exercise.[1] Intense exercise, in which you work at over seventy-five percent of your maximum aerobic capacity, can deplete the working muscles' glycogen reserves in as little as an hour or two, depending on how fit you are and on your prior glycogen reserves.[2]

The body also burns fat for energy, but not as efficiently. As muscle glycogen is depleted, the liver contributes some of its reserves, but if you continue to exercise intensely, the liver may be unable to keep pace, and you may feel the effects of a sharp drop in your blood sugar level. If this happens, your muscles simply 'give out' and you experience extreme exhaustion. At the same time the glucose deprivation in your brain and nervous system may make you confused or disoriented.[3] The result of a high-intensity workout may leave you feeling exhausted and famished. It is common in such a situation to overeat in order to replenish glucose stores.

For example, if you increase the resistance on an exercise bicycle to get a better workout this can result in increased stress not only on the knee joints but also on the soles of the feet. Pedalling hard with few revolutions per minute can make it difficult for oxygen to reach the muscles, especially if you are not a conditioned cyclist. In addition, increased metabolic demands may promote a build-up of lactic acid, a factor in muscle pain and fatigue. Draining your energy will not help you establish a better lifestyle.

Activity could be part of your lifestyle change and not just the means to losing weight. Increasing physical activity until you lose weight is parallel to going on a diet until you lose weight. If a lifestyle change isn't in place and the enjoyment isn't there, you will stop exercising and go off the diet. The result is short-term success and a sense of failure when the weight returns.

Myth 2: Exercising only until you lose weight

'I'm going to the fitness class six times a week and I'm losing inches. I can't wait till I reach my goal weight so that I can stop exercising.' Unfortunately this person found exercising stressful and didn't know that if you start and stop exercise, you can increase body weight. In fact, animal studies have shown that cessation of exercise can lead to increased body fat later. So if you treat exercise only as a method to lose weight you run the risk of actually making your body fatter.

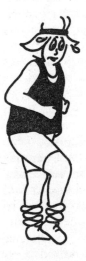

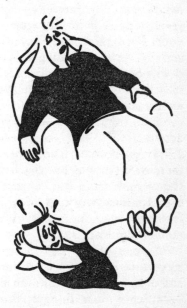

Studies have shown that making activity part of your lifestyle change is a more effective way of losing weight in the long run. Aim for a gradual increase in activity that becomes part of your daily routine. Lower intensity, longer duration types of activity are more likely to become part of your lifestyle. These activities will eventually become habit, but it will take time. Enjoying the process eliminates the desire to stop.

In order to allow yourself to 'get hooked' on exercise, be aware of how you feel and how your body reacts before and after exercising. After exercising regularly (i.e. every second day) for a few weeks, try skipping a week and find out if you miss it. The feeling of energy, vitality, and exhilaration that you get from regular activity may make you want to continue. Endorphins, a chemical released while exercising, serve as a natural tranquilliser that soothes both the body and mind. Once you experience the internal benefits of activity, it is difficult to do without it.

Myth 3: Exercising vigorously burns more fat
Higher intensity activity burns more carbohydrates than fat.[4] In the first twelve to thirty minutes of activity, you use up mainly carbohydrates as your fuel source.[5,6] This means that your body will be drawing from the carbohydrate stores in your liver (glycogen stores). Engaging in higher intensity activity such as jogging or running is hard on the knees and does not build up endurance if you continue the jogging for only a short period of time. With vigorous exercise you are not giving your body a chance to switch over to using more fat as the fuel source. This occurs only after about thirty minutes of activity.

As you become fitter, the training effect will allow you to increase the use of fat as a fuel source.[7] Running may wear off the calories more quickly and for this reason burn more total fat. However, working at this higher intensity level may reduce the duration of the activity. In this way, the benefits of sustained activity are lost.[8] People who do aerobics at a higher intensity level are often starved after a workout. They may have burned more total calories which used up some of their carbohydrate stores and caused some burning of fat as their fuel source. But because of their hunger and eating after the workout they replenished their glycogen stores and minimised the burning of fat. The lesson here is that you can:

- work at a level that is comfortable for you where you can sustain the activity for a longer period of time rather than engage in short bursts of activity;

- increase your intensity gradually as you become fitter;

- use an activity you enjoy that leaves you feeling energised not exhausted, and tune into how you feel before and after your activity with regard to energy level and appetite control; and

- work at a level that controls your appetite rather than leaves you feeling famished. (Even if you do eat a little more due to activity, there will still be a net loss of energy expended. Remember to replenish your fluids first to rehydrate any fluid lost. You may actually be thirsty and not hungry.)

Karen, her mother, and her sister went for a walk. The mother walked with her arms flinging, racing to get to her destination. 'It doesn't do any good unless you walk briskly,' she said, as she huffed and puffed to keep her pace. 'I want to lose five pounds by next week.' At the end she was exhausted and had not enjoyed the walk or the scenery. Her focus was the destination, not the journey. Karen walked at a comfortable rate, and was still able to talk to her sister. Her heart rate was going up, but not racing, so she felt both physically and psychologically refreshed at the end of the walk. In fact, she enjoyed it so much that she made this a habit. Each time she walked, it became easier to walk slightly more quickly and still feel comfortable. She was gradually becoming fitter and she revelled in the experience.

Like many people coming into the programme, Janice was jogging regularly to lose weight. She felt tired because jogging was hard on her body. She was thrilled to hear that walking was more effective for weight loss due to its lower intensity and she enjoyed the activity much more. She noted how walking helped her to stabilise her weight. Another client commented, 'I tried to fit jogging in. What a relief to find I can enjoy walking at lunchtime with a friend and it's okay!'

Comparison of impact forces being generated and delivered to the lower body

WALKING   one times your body weight

RUNNING   three times your body weight

JUMPING   up to ten times your body weight

Walking at a comfortable speed may increase the heart rate forty to fifty percent above the normal heart rate. This is more than enough to stimulate the lungs and heart and increase oxygen uptake and delivery to all body tissues. According to experts in the field of exercise physiology, two-and-a-half miles (four km) of walking will produce the same aerobic benefits as five miles (eight km) of bicycling, one quarter of a mile (0.4 km) of swimming, or one mile (1.6 km) of running.

It is interesting to note that it is often Type A personalities – the hard-working, aggressive, competitive individuals – who choose jogging or competitive sports because they think that aggressive activities will lessen their chance of heart disease. However, instead of running off their aggression and tension, they actually run into it and increase their chances of developing heart disease above the twenty-five percent chance they already have due to their personality type.

Myth 4: Activity burns only calories
Regular activity provides more benefits to your health than simply burning calories. It revs up your system from four to six hours after the completion of the activity.[9] It gives you the energy to meet everyday and emergency requirements, and to effectively use and enjoy leisure time. What matters is not how many calories you use up during the activity but how much you increase your metabolic rate and then keep it going at this faster rate even when the activity is completed. This is why regular activity as part of your lifestyle is important.

For example, if you exercise from 8:00 to 8:30 in the morning, your body will continue to burn calories at a faster rate than if you had not taken any exercise. The increase in metabolic rate is caused by the demand for energy for muscle building and repair resulting from exercise, providing that the exercise is of an appropriate intensity and duration. If you work at the level that is comfortable for you it will allow activity to control rather than increase your appetite.

Regular activity gives you sustained energy. Gradually increase your activity so that you can participate in the activity at least every second day in order to derive the maximum benefit. Start more slowly if you wish. As the activity becomes a lifestyle change, you will eventually choose to do it more frequently. Let it happen naturally. If you think it is difficult to take time for an activity in terms of a half hour off from your daily routine, keep in mind that you will get back that time and more in terms of your increased efficiency and energy level, which will allow you to accomplish more in less time.

THE PERKS OF PHYSICAL ACTIVITY

Exercise and obesity
According to experts, exercise may carry important benefits for the large person even in the absence of weight loss. In sufficient amounts, physical activity can improve nearly every negative consequence of obesity.[10,11]

Improves self-image
Being fat in a weight-conscious society can undermine self-esteem. Yet some studies have shown that large men and women in physical training programmes exhibit marked improvement in self-satisfaction, self-acceptance, and a sense of personal worth. A Harris poll in 1979 found that physically active people reported more self-confidence, a better self-image, and greater psychological wellbeing than inactive people.

Control over one's life – the ability to make choices – is vital for a positive self-image and a feeling of personal power. A renewed sense of control is experienced after a period of regular activity, which facilitates the ability to resolve problems of personal dissatisfaction and poor body image.

The body adapts to the demands of physical exertion by increasing muscular strength and endurance, whereas long periods of food restriction produce diminishing returns, and increase both physical and psychological stress. During periods of increased stress, feelings of lethargy often result, with the release of adrenalin and cortisol, both stress-related hormones. These hormones are metabolised by exercise, which decreases their undesirable effect. Long-term activities also result in the secretion of endorphins by the brain. These small, morphine-like substances can produce a feeling of exhilaration, which reduces stress and, through a complex process, may even reduce fat storage.

The improved self-image and sense of accomplishment resulting from exercise may be instrumental in the development of long-term lifestyle changes that lead to permanent weight control and a healthier life. For health, walk tall with shoulders back, pelvis forward and bum tucked in.

Depresses mood swings
During physical activity, the release of endorphins acts as a pain killer and tranquilliser making you feel more relaxed. Eating and laughter can also release this chemical. Changing your attitude and your lifestyle by adopting a more light-hearted approach can make you happier and healthier. The same temporary 'high' that you get from eating can be transferred to a more sustained 'high' from activity.

Making that special time for yourself
Physical activity can serve as a release valve for stress and give you the time to think things through.

Improve self-esteem
With lifestyle changes you will notice health benefits within a few months and feel a sense of accomplishment. Activity can help you to channel your energy inward to deal with inner problems.

Physical activity regulates appetite
Sedentary people who do little activity may overeat because their appetite control mechanism is not functioning properly. The stomach is not sending a signal to the brain when they are full. Exercise at a proper intensity puts this back into balance.

Deanna was tuned into her body with regard to food and ate

till she was satisfied; she felt that she was not overeating. If her eyes were bigger than her stomach and she overloaded her plate, she would eat until she was full, and then leave the rest on her plate. This was quite an accomplishment for her. She had lost weight and it had stabilised. But even though she was following her internal hunger signals, she seemed to be gaining back some weight. In this case, she was no longer active and tended to be in a constant 'rush' with her new job. Some of this rushed feeling transferred to her eating and she was able to eat more before her stomach signalled to her brain that she was full. Without activity, her appetite control mechanism was not working properly and so she may have been taking in more food before she was satisfied. Keep in mind that activity, done at an intensity appropriate for you, can regulate your appetite.

Physical activity keeps you fit
Activity improves joint problems and decreases muscle cramps. Drinking sufficient water also helps to lessen muscle cramps.

Physical activity lowers blood pressure
Blood pressure is the force of blood pushing against the walls of the arteries as it flows through them. Physical activity lowers blood pressure in three ways. First, it aids in the loss of body fat. For every extra pound of body fat you need an extra mile of blood vessels to nourish it. Second, it tones the blood vessels to make them more elastic. Third, exercise reduces the deposition of fat on the artery walls, preventing the opening from becoming smaller. A larger opening requires less pressure against the artery walls. The bonus is that as you become more fit, your heart becomes stronger. With each contraction, it pushes more blood to the rest of the body.

Physical activity lowers blood sugar levels
With exercise the immediate rise in blood sugar levels after a meal is less pronounced, and sugar is released in smaller doses. This is accomplished by increasing sensitivity to the cell receptors, so that the insulin can allow blood sugar to enter cells more readily. The blood sugar is released into the bloodstream at a slower, more gradual rate, providing a more steady supply of energy.

Eating properly, coupled with activity, allows you to feel more energetic. This is partly due to blood sugar control. Even if you do not have diabetes, poor eating habits may lead to erratic blood sugar control. For example, twenty-four-year-old Brenda was not overweight but had poor, erratic eating habits. She was always tired and lived on cake and little food. Blood tests indicated that Brenda had hypoglycaemia (low blood sugar level). When Brenda established a regular eating pattern balancing both carbohydrate and protein sources, she had the energy to become more active, which in turn gave her more energy. She became more efficient and productive. It's a matter of balance!

Physical activity improves circulation
Physical activity adds to an increased energy level as oxygen and nutrients are carried throughout the body more efficiently.

Physical activity improves digestion
You will find that constipation decreases as the natural movement of the intestine is improved.

Myth 5: The same exercise every day is necessary
Some people think that doing the same type of exercise activity every day is necessary. Rather, cross-training for a more balanced body is preferable. Alternating the type of activities done on a daily basis gives specific muscles a chance to relax. For example, walking on one day and rowing another day uses different muscles. Cross-training allows you to exercise more muscle groups than a single activity would do. For instance, cycling builds your lower body, and rowing works your upper body, so alternating them can help give you the benefits of both while you build aerobic endurance. It also minimises the stress felt from always using the same muscles and joints.

Allowing your muscles to rest and using other muscles reduces the risk of injury. Better muscle balance is also achieved. For example, walking or running strengthens the hamstring muscles (located at the rear of the thigh) more than it does the quadriceps at the front of the thigh. This muscle imbalance may lead to injury. By adding cycling on alternate days (which strengthens the quadriceps) you can work complementary muscle groups in your legs and thus achieve better muscle balance.[12]

Vary the types of exercise you do. People in long-term aerobic programmes strengthen their hearts and typically build up their leg muscles, but may lose muscle mass in their upper body. To balance your exercise programme, use your own body weight as resistance in push-ups, sit-ups, and pull-ups. There's no set amount of weight you should lift and no standard against which you should measure yourself: the goal is to work out according to your capabilities.[13]

Myth 6: Eat little, exercise a lot for weight loss
The type of activity rather than the amount of activity is what counts. Restrictive eating (dieting) combined with frequent physical activity will cause you to drain your protein or muscle tissue if insufficient carbohydrates are consumed. If your calories consumption is too low to supply your energy needs, your body then breaks down valuable protein tissue to use for energy. With the breakdown of protein, your metabolic rate is further decreased.

Many diets are low in carbohydrates. Remember that, regardless of the intensity of the activity, in the first thirty minutes carbohydrates are the main fuel source. They break down into glucose, which provides you with energy. If insufficient bread, cereals, potatoes, rice, and pasta are consumed muscle protein will be broken down into glucose.[14] Exercise preserves lean muscle tissue only if sufficient calories are consumed, including carbohydrates.[15]

Between the ages of thirty and seventy the average person loses thirty to forty percent of the body's muscle mass. Exercise can retard these changes for as long as twenty years.[16]

Myth 7: Exercise increases appetite
Exercising at a higher intensity depletes your glycogen stores faster, leaving you with a lower blood sugar level. The result is that instead of activity controlling your appetite, it may actually increase it. Lower intensity activity will draw less from your glycogen stores and allow you to sustain the activity for a longer period of time. Tune into your body and decide on the level that is right for you. You can increase your heart rate and still be able

to carry on a conversation with a friend. Putting an extra strain on your body with stressful activity gives no added benefit. You should feel energised, not exhausted and famished, after exercise.

Myth 8: Exercise is boring

Taking on an exercise programme and giving it up just as quickly produces the same short-term gain as a quick weight-loss diet. The extra physical strain that comes from exercising above your capacity or eating below your basic needs leaves you in a weakened condition. Having fun with activity will ensure that you are doing what your body can endure. Choose something you enjoy and learn to work at your own level. If you do not like aerobics, find a programme or activity that interests you. Don't participate only because your best friend is doing it.

Exercise is a skill. Once developed it is difficult to do without it. It becomes part of you and when it's fun it's something that you look forward to. As June says, 'I discovered swimming and it's great. I feel so invigorated.'

A positive attitude is also necessary. Once on a cross-country ski-trip, I had to go down a small hill. I froze. I couldn't face this challenge. In my mind, I felt that I could not do it, and so the self-fulfilling prophecy came true as I went down the hill on my bum. I didn't even give myself a chance to fall down or fail. I got it over with, not allowing myself to experience the exhilaration of trying.

Contemplating this and becoming more comfortable with skiing, I tried to develop a positive 'I-can-do-it' attitude. I did it gradually, stopping partway to decrease my fear of speed. I fell from time to time but I also made more hills with my skis in place. Best of all, I allowed myself to enjoy the whole experience. Focusing on the fun and the improvement of self rather than on the competition keep you going. So many of us fail because we feel we aren't good enough to compete, so we don't exercise at all. If you have a positive attitude and find an activity that you enjoy, you will keep coming back.

Kevin was anxious every time he had to play football. His father always concentrated on winning. Eventually Kevin found excuses to stop playing and began watching more television. At least this was non-threatening. On the other hand, Tim's father's attitude towards fitness emphasised fun. He practised with his son so that he would feel more confident with the ball. The sport became an enjoyable event that kept him active, and Tim continued to include activity as part of his daily routine as he got older.

Myth 9: Exercise plus dieting increases metabolic rate
Physical activity increases the metabolic rate about ten percent which may offset some of the fifteen to thirty percent decrease in metabolic rate when dieting. However, the net increase in metabolic rate is still five to twenty percent.[17,18] The answer, of course, is to stop dieting. Focus instead on healthier eating by gradually changing the type of foods you are consuming. There may not be a great difference in the total number of calories eaten but the type of calories will change, and this is important. By avoiding a marked drop in calorie intake your body will have a chance to adjust to the gradual change. Gradual is the key. Then the body won't be fooled into dropping the metabolic rate to protect you from starvation since you are not drastically cutting calories but maintaining them at close to the original level. Remember, it is not the quantity but the types of foods consumed that contribute to weight gain.

Initially when teaching the programme, I noticed that clients dropped the fat content of their meals quickly when they realised that it was these calories that contributed to weight gain (more about this in Chapters 4 and 5). Many lost weight more quickly but did not give their systems a chance to adjust either physically (with regard to metabolic rate) or psychologically (change in taste) to the sudden change. If you do this the result is quicker weight loss which inevitably results in quicker weight gain. YCCD aims to help you escape from this all-or-nothing mentality.

Myth 10: Exercise causes you to lose weight on the scales
Without activity, only fifty percent of weight lost is fat. Muscle cannot be stored in a dry form; it is stored with water. This makes muscle weigh more than fat. Therefore, an increase in muscle mass may mean inches lost, but not necessarily weight lost. This is another indication of why the scales do not count.

An increase in muscle mass results in an increase in metabolic rate. Muscle tissue burns more calories at rest than fat does. Men, whose body composition consists of more muscle mass, burn more calories at rest. Frequent dieting can result in weight loss, including muscle mass. Unfortunately, once the weight is regained, it is mostly fat. Exercise provides an opportunity to rebuild muscle tissue that is vital to your health and wellbeing.

Myth 11: Sit-ups get rid of fat in the stomach area

Spot reducing tones, but it does not get rid of fat in the area you are working on. Results from products that claim to do this are only temporary. The gut buster, toning clinics, and new gadgets to rid you of that 'paunch' are not the answer. These fads in the exercise field are comparable to fad diets. They work temporarily, and some may shed inches, but often at the expense of health. Poor techniques may result in back problems. Fat loss does not occur. These methods merely tone by making muscles more taut and helping with body alignment. They certainly do not improve your health or make you fitter.

Body builders work out with weights. They want to display muscle tone but since abdominal muscles, for example, are beneath fat they must get rid of the fat. The body builder or weight trainer may look fit but his endurance may be poor. In order for the weight trainer to lift weights, he needs the stamina that comes from improving heart–lung functions of the cardiovascular system. The weight lifter may be strong, but does he exude inner health?

Doing sit-ups helps with alignment and toning only by making muscles tighter. While strong abdominal muscles provide better support for the back, in order to get rid of the fat some form of aerobic activity is necessary. Lifting weights can help to increase muscle mass which indirectly will increase metabolic rate due to the change in body composition. However, for sustained energy and fat loss to occur, aerobic activity is the answer. Aim for the balance in different types of activity to achieve the right combination for you!

Myth 12: Exercise takes time

If you make physical activity important enough in your life to give it priority, the regular activity will give you the added benefit of increased energy levels and improved efficiency. By accomplishing tasks in less time, exercise actually gives you time back, rather than taking time away from your daily routine.

HOW TO MAKE AN EXERCISE PROGRAMME WORK FOR YOU

If you exercise consistently and regularly at a lower intensity level you will develop a training effect. The result is an increased capacity to work with less effort due to the glycogen-sparing effect of using more fat as the fuel source. If you do this you will not get tired as quickly because you preserve carbohydrate stores that supply you with continued energy. However, it is important to keep up the exercise. This adaptation or training effect will be lost within three or more days of inactivity.[19]

Exercising at too high a level for your body to feel comfortable can result in heavier breathing or feeling out of breath. This indicates that you are no longer using oxygen, and are switching over to anaerobic activity. This leads to a build-up of lactic acid causing muscle fatigue. There is absolutely no advantage in pushing yourself to work at this high level.

Work on changing past negative experiences that you may have had with exercising into positive activities that are enjoyable, interesting, safe, and meaningful to you. To keep the activity you choose safe, it is important to develop a warm-up, aerobic, and cool-down routine, even for walking. Exercise for energy, not exhaustion. If you are tired after exercising and sore, you are exercising at too high a limit. Pay attention to your body. Do you feel your heart rate increasing, yet you can still carry on a conversation? This is the level that is right for you.

Warm-up
Purpose:

- to stretch, loosen up, and relax muscles;
- to prevent injury;
- to stimulate circulation; and
- to prepare you physically and psychologically for the workout.

Warming up your body takes only five or ten minutes and can be compared to warming up the engine of your car. If you turn on the ignition and don't take time to warm it up on a cold day, you may do some harm to the engine. Usually the car tells you to take a little longer to warm it up by stalling as you start to drive. If you do not take the time to warm up your body, you may harm it as well. Walking slowly, doing some stretches to prepare your muscles, or partaking in the activity of your choice at a slower pace warms up your body.

I like the game of tennis. I used to go on the court and start to play vigorously almost right away, not having the patience to take the time to warm up. I ended up running for the ball a lot and was not systematic in my approach. These days, I warm up my muscles first by doing a few shoulder rolls, stretching out my calves, bouncing the ball against my racket, then rallying slowly at first. I am taking it slowly, gradually, and building up to a level that is comfortable for me.

My tennis game has improved because my body is more focused on what I am doing. Instead of rushing to get the ball and stopping cold, and in many cases missing it, I pace myself better and have more rhythm to my steps. I also focus on the ball and what I am doing which helps improve my game. I can now take this more methodical approach because I have the energy to think clearly. I am no longer trying to wear myself out in the first few minutes. Best of all, I enjoy tennis more as well as the process of gradually improving.

Aerobic Portion
Purpose:

● improve heart–lung function (cardiovascular benefits).

An acrobic activity is any exercise that increases the body's intake and use of oxygen, The exercise does this by increasing the heartbeat, within prudent limits, and improving the heart–lung action. The adequacy of your oxygen supply depends on how much you take in by breathing, and how efficiently the blood distributes it throughout the body. To be aerobic, exercise must be active and sustained, enough to cause you to breathe more deeply and more often. If you aim, with your aerobic exercise programme, to be slightly to moderately out of breath, the benefits are that you will burn more fat as a fuel source, you will have the ability to carry on the activity for a longer period of time, and your cardiovascular system will work better to make you fitter as well. Try to maintain aerobic activity for about twenty minutes. This will increase your heart rate, causing more efficient blood circulation.

In the target heart rate zone this is presented as the sixty-five to seventy percent range where maximum heart rate is calculated by using the following formula: 220 minus person's age. For example, for a forty-five-year-old woman, the maximum heart rate is equal to $220 - 45 = 175$. 65% of $175 = 114$ beats/min. $(0.65 \times 175) = 19$ beats/10 sec. This gives the range of sixty-five percent of maximum heart rate at which this woman needs to be working when in the aerobic zone. This range will allow enjoyment of the activity while participating in it, and will allow the activity to be sustained in order to derive the benefits from it.

Your heart is a muscle. When you work it you strengthen it. With a strengthened heart, each contraction pumps more blood throughout the body, thus making it more efficient. With efficiency, your heart does not have to work as hard to achieve the same effect. Compare the effort it takes to walk up two or three flights of stairs before and after three months of training. As you become fitter your heart rate at rest in the morning will be lower because your heart will not have to work as hard to achieve the same effect.

AGE	Target Heart Rate Zone
20	22–23 beats/10 sec.
30	20–22 beats/10 sec.
40	19–21 beats/10 sec.
50	18–20 beats/10 sec.
60	17–19 beats/10 sec.
70	16–18 beats/10 sec.

The purpose of including target heart rate zones here is merely to familiarise you with them. You will see them in fitness clubs; however, this programme is related to fitness and lifestyle rather than to a number on the chart. Learn to tune into working at the level where you feel your heart rate coming up, but are still able to carry on a conversation. This is the right intensity for you. Aim to feel energised rather than exhausted at the end of your fitness break. Including warm-ups and cool-downs, listening to your body, and participating in an activity that you enjoy will help you to achieve this goal.

Cool-down
Purpose:

- to allow heart rate to gradually return to normal;
- to stretch and relax all body muscles;
- to reduce the chance of pain or injury to muscles; and
- to prevent the possibility of sore muscles later on.

Once again compare your body to a car. When you are driving quickly at sixty miles (100 km) per hour and you are coming to a traffic light, you slow down gradually rather than slam on the brake. The same applies to your body. You don't want to get going at full speed and then come to an abrupt stop. The result will be fatigue and sore muscles the next day. After exercise your muscles are warm. It's a perfect time to stretch them out and increase your flexibility. Cooling down takes five to ten minutes and may involve working the same large muscle groups as you did for the warm-up, walking slowly, or partaking in the activity slowly. Going full speed to come home and flop in the chair is not enforcing a lifestyle change. If you make it fun and enjoyable, you will derive more energy from the activity. Listen to your body!

Any of these different activities will help you make fitness into a lifestyle change that you can enjoy for a lifetime:

CYCLING

Work up a faster cycling rate and heart rate without the tension on the bike. Using the tension will work your leg muscles but you won't derive the aerobic benefit. Increasing the tension on the bicycle will also tire your legs more quickly so that you may not be able to sustain the activity over the required period of time.

GOLF

Walking around the course rather than using the motorised cart is beneficial. Formerly, it was thought that this type of activity was 'stop and go' and would not allow your heart rate to stay in the target heart rate zone for the required period of time to derive the cardiovascular benefit. But the aim of a more active lifestyle is achieved with this activity. It also creates a good balance in lifestyle.

ROWING

This activity uses the arm muscles and is a good complement to walking. Be gradual and consistent rather than racing and then doing nothing. Pace yourself.

TENNIS

The aerobic benefit can be derived from this activity if you pace yourself rather than undergoing the more fanatic 'stop and go' method of playing tennis.

AEROBICS

For maximum benefit find a fitness routine that incorporates lifestyle moves and fun. Be sure to include warm-up, aerobic, and cool-down in the routine. Many routines also include a mat portion that helps you with strength and flexibility. Ensure that the atmosphere allows you to work at the level at which you feel comfortable and that you do not come away feeling sore or stiff.

Safe techniques are crucial so that you do not injure your body. We have a fitness video specifically geared to people who are not used to regular activity, and aimed at fun. These lifestyle moves can help you with your everyday life. The safe techniques are designed to reduce the chance of injury. For more help in this area, see the order form at the end of this book.

WALKING

The best and safest exercise for people of any age is walking. It is:

- safe and efficient;
- can be followed throughout life;
- strengthens bones and organs including the heart;
- improves many body functions especially blood circulation, digestion, and elimination (stimulates contractions of the intestine, helping to push food through);
- lubricates the joints, reducing the pain of arthritis;
- lowers high blood pressure and reduces the risk of heart attack and strokes by improving cardiovascular function;
- helps to relive pain from varicose veins;
- is the least likely activity to cause any muscle, joint, or bone injury; and
- has these other benefits of regular activity (helps you sleep better, reduces tension and related headaches, relieves depression, improves emotional health, sharpens the senses, increases mental alertness, helps maintain a youthful outlook).

As a lifestyle change, walking does not mean just going out for a walk every day or second day. It could also include taking every opportunity to walk during the day as well.

HELPFUL HINTS

Use the stairs instead of a lift or escalator where appropriate. At airports, hotels, shopping centres use the stairs or walk up or down the escalator. An interesting study found that merely climbing five flights of stairs or walking more than five blocks daily reduced the incidence of heart attack by twenty-five percent.[20]

Park your car a little further away and walk the rest of the way. This will also save you from the congestion in the car park at the end of the day. When friends come over try going for a walk instead of engaging in conversation while sitting and eating. There is nothing like scenery to stimulate exciting conversation. Plan vacations to include your new lifestyle of increased activity. A more active lifestyle becomes a way of life; it is not simply something that you turn on and off. It may take some time to internalise it and make it part of your inner being, but eventually it will be as routine as brushing your teeth. You won't feel right if you don't have a walk during the day. Remember that walking a mile burns ten to twenty percent fewer calories than jogging a mile, though obviously it takes longer. If you walk briskly, you can obtain nearly the same aerobic benefits provided by running.

Physical activity allows you to think more clearly, be more efficient, have a happier disposition, and renew energy to allow you to accomplish more in less time. The result is that you have more free time to do the things you really want to do.

Remember to replace fluids lost through exercise. Physical exercise without fluid replacement enhances crystallisation of both calcium oxalate and uric acid, largely as a result of reduced urine output and acid in the urine. If you do not drink enough fluids, your body protects you from becoming dehydrated by reducing the amount of fluid you excrete in the form of urine. The more concentrated urine, noticeable by its darker colour, increases the chance of formation of kidney stones. Increase fluid intake during physical activity to compensate for sweat loss.[21]

If you lose a few pounds of weight after exercising, this is water loss in the form of sweat. Replenish your fluid intake to bring you back to your original weight prior to exercise. Another indication of rehydration is the lighter colour of your urine. Keep in mind that taking vitamin pills may make your urine darker so that you may mistake it for a state of dehydration.

GETTING HOOKED ON ACTIVITY

Computers and modern technology make your life easier, and so you are less likely to have an active lifestyle. Children are growing up using less and less of their muscle capacity. Playing football or running around are being replaced by sitting comfortably on a tyre and being pulled by a speedboat, plying computer games, or working radio-controlled machines or airplanes. If you continue to do this you will lose your energy and vitality. How can you break this cycle and increase your leisure-time physical activity? You could plan more active holidays and get involved in more sports.

Many of us live a fast-paced lifestyle. We work out because it's good for us, not because we enjoy it. Since we work intensely we tend to work out intensely. It's difficult to enjoy physical activity with this approach. On the other hand, many people become addicted to exercise and suffer from withdrawal pains when they are deprived. They exhibit the same dependence on exercise as dieters do on diets. These individuals exercise as an end in itself rather than as a means to physical fitness. Some of them cannot stop exercising, even when their muscles and joints have become seriously injured. The symptoms of exercise addicts are:

- needing to run or exercise daily to maintain a basic level of functioning;

- expressing minor withdrawal symptoms, such as irritability, guilt, or anxiety, when unable to exercise for a day or two; experiencing major withdrawal symptoms, such as depression, loss of self-esteem, or lack of interest in other activities when unable to exercise for longer periods of time;

- exercising even against medical advice;

- risking physical injury;

- organising life around exercise;

- putting exercise above everything else, including job or relationships; and

- striving for greater achievement.

Intense commitment to exercise as a means in itself cannot have long-term benefits. You cannot hurry to be fit or stop when you reach your goal. Exercising for the wrong reasons won't help you to adopt exercise as a permanent part of your lifestyle.

The good news is that recent studies show that even mild physical activity is helpful in counteracting the effects of an unhealthy way of eating or in lowering cholesterol and high blood pressure. So if you have been laughing at your neighbours as they garden or rake leaves (lifestyle moves) while you are riding your stationary bike that goes nowhere, take a second look at who is getting hooked on an active lifestyle. Observe the enjoyment they get from living a more active lifestyle.

In the past twenty years the fitness movement has been focusing too much on performance that stresses the importance of doing more. When you change your focus to overall fitness and wellbeing and redefine success, you will realise that you can improve your health by doing those simple chores around the house or even taking a leisurely stroll. Regular physical activity protects you against heart disease. Even if you are not working out to a point that brings your heart rate up to the target heart rate, you will still benefit.

Ellen's speed-walking left her husband Ron tired when he tried to keep up, causing his enthusiasm to wane. Ron, who weighs 330 pounds, was determined to work at his own level. Now he feels good after walking instead of ending up 'pooped' and with sore legs. 'This is for life,' he says to Ellen, 'and it will take time for me to comfortably work up to your level, so go on ahead of me.'

Remember that exercising above your comfort level in an effort to get fit too quickly will make you feel exhausted and will make it difficult for you to transfer from an inactive to an active state. Develop a positive rather than a negative attitude towards activity and the rest will follow. Find an activity that you enjoy. Work at your own level and increase the amount of activity time gradually. Stick with it!

Regularity is the key for exercise, and if you don't enjoy the type or intensity level of the activity then the activity may be short-lived. Your memory of the activity should be one of enjoyment. When you stop exercising, you lose the beneficial effects of exercise. This process is known as detraining. How quickly this occurs depends on how fit you are and how long you have been exercising or how long you have been sedentary.

In a study done at Washington University School of Medicine in St Louis, runners, cyclists, and swimmers who had worked out regularly and vigorously for years abstained from exercise. After twelve weeks they lost more than half their gains in aerobic conditioning compared to a sedentary control group who hadn't exercised regularly for at least eight years.

In another study, sedentary people undertook an eight-week cycling regime and then stopped for eight weeks. The result was that all their aerobic gains were lost. They returned to their pretraining fitness levels. Cutting back on exercise is less devastating than stopping exercise. Studies show that these people are often able to avoid or postpone the effects of detraining.[22]

Lifestyle activities (walking or climbing stairs) that are done regularly can help you become fit while enjoying it.

A recent report in the *Journal of the American Medical Association* studied more than 13,000 people for an average of eight years to analyse the effects of fitness on longevity. Five groups of people were divided according to fitness levels. The least-fit group who were also the most sedentary had the highest mortality rates by far. The big surprise was that the death rate dropped most sharply in the second least-fit group, by sixty percent for men and forty-eight percent for women.[23]

Researchers estimated that a person need only walk briskly for thirty to sixty minutes every day to be in this group. The three fittest groups, including people who jogged up to forty miles a week, derived relatively small additional benefits from their exercise. Why kill yourself to maintain a gruelling schedule when in fact you don't have to be a marathon runner to greatly reduce your risks of heart or other disease? Modest increases in lower intensity activities such as brisk walking will probably add years to your life. So why not take opportunities to use the stairs or go for a walk? Build up the strength of your heart and enhance your level of active living.

As you gradually make modest improvements in aerobic fitness, the calories expended will increase the high density lipoprotein (HDL) that will protect you against heart disease. Here is an example of daily leisure-time activities that will expend an average of 200 calories a day.

MONDAY	Walk	40 min =	140 cal
	Stairs at work	10 min =	80 cal
TUESDAY	Stairs at work	10 min =	80 cal
WEDNESDAY	Walk	30 min =	100 cal
	Rake lawn	40 min =	160 cal
	Stairs at work	5 min =	40 cal
THURSDAY	Stairs at work	10 min =	80 cal
FRIDAY	Walk	60 min =	200 cal
	Stairs at work	10 min =	80 cal
SATURDAY	Mow yard	60 min =	300 cal
	Dancing	60 min =	330 cal
SUNDAY	Walk with family	60 min =	200 cal
	TOTAL		*= 1790 cal*

The good news is that all that is needed to significantly prolong life is a moderate level of activity. This fact applies regardless of the presence of other risk factors such as cholesterol levels, blood pressure, body composition, cigarette smoking, or family medical history. According to Dr Steven Blair, one of the physicians conducting the study, the men were better off to have high cholesterol and be fit, than to have low cholesterol and be in a low fitness category.

Another study of 17,000 Harvard alumni found that exercise levels to use 2000 calories a week through day-to-day activities such as walking, stair climbing, and light sports such as golf, afforded significant protection from heart disease.[24] This maximum protective effect of a sixty-four percent reduction in risk of heart disease was reached by including leisure-time physical activities as seen in the table (p93). It is interesting to note that if you exceed 2000 calories per week in leisure-time physical activities you gain little further benefit; in fact, you increase the risk of orthopaedic injury.

Boredom can make you feel lazy and tricks you into thinking you're physically tired. It catches all of us if we don't watch out, so fight back by finding an activity you really enjoy and stick with it. If you tried an activity and you didn't care for it, try it again with your new attitude towards activity. When I was first introduced to golf I went to the driving range, took a few lessons, and tried my hand at the golf course. But I just couldn't get interested in trying to shoot this small ball into the hole. So I gave up and never considered trying again. One day, a friend took me for lunch overlooking a beautiful golf course. It was lovely, but I never considered trying golf again until she presented me with a new perspective. 'Golf is an excuse to walk in a really nice park,' she said. 'We don't even keep score, Linda.'

We often feel that we have to be good at an activity in order to enjoy it. Yet the very act of participating in an invigorating, natural, and stimulating environment can be enjoyable in itself. Observe those around you who enjoy the internal benefits of active living. The next time you go to a social event where there is dancing, try staying on the dance floor for at least twenty minutes and just keep dancing. Feel the music and enjoy yourself! Remember to stop every half hour or so to drink water, whether you feel thirsty or not. Proper hydration keeps you going but too much alcohol will dehydrate you and make you feel sleepy.

Enjoyable occasions allow you to build in some special time for yourself while being more active in a creative way. Find more opportunities to 'kick up your heels' and enjoy yourself while gradually increasing your level of activity.

ACTION POINTS

● Increase physical activities into your present lifestyle, e.g. walking up stairs, parking further away from your destination, gardening, walking or cycling instead of using the car/bus.

● Create time for additional activities that you think you may enjoy and can sustain, e.g. swimming, tennis, dancing, gym, walking.

● Gain confidence from activities you enjoy, then experiment with new activities. Keep those you enjoy.

Listen to your body to see how you feel in body and mind before and after participating in an activity. This will help you to want to do it again.

Let exercise become your leisure time and participate at a level that is comfortable for your body. The diet mentality will cause you to overexercise or punish yourself with exercise. Catch this way of thinking and turn it around.

Exercise for energy, not exhaustion. If you are tired after exercising and sore, you are exercising at too high a level.

Increase the amount of activity one step at a time.

Notice how you feel when you warm up and cool down before and after exercise. Are you less likely to be stiff and sore the next day? Notice the difference.

Enjoy the lasting effects if you stick with it!

4

Healthy Eating

Balance your meals to fill your needs for
fullness and energy. Eat regularly starting
with a balanced breakfast.

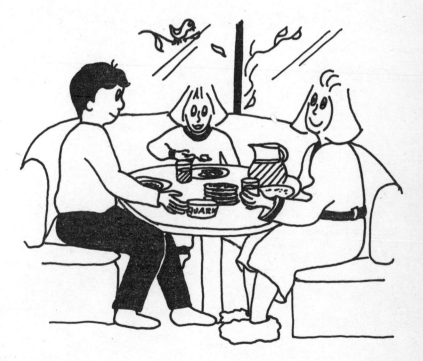

Part of the balance in the quality of life includes healthy eating. Most of us eat out more often these days. Even the meals eaten at home are not the tasty home-cooked kind but are the quick-to-prepare kind because of our busy lifestyles.

Yet healthy eating is important and it is the next step in giving you more energy to focus on your road to health. Don't worry, that doesn't mean eating salads and fruits alone. That would only set you up to binge. After all, it's human nature to want something that you can't have.

If you've been dieting, that will put you out of tune with your body and its signals of hunger and fullness. You must begin by eating regularly, starting with breakfast, in order to tune back in. One of my clients felt that when she started to eat breakfast, it made her more hungry by lunch time and she began to eat more frequently; whereas formerly she did not eat all day until supper. It takes three to four hours to digest a balanced breakfast, so you will be hungry by lunch. If you eat these meals and stop eating when you are full you will ultimately eat less at supper time and throughout the evening. Once you get 'hooked' on eating breakfast, your body will find it difficult to do without it.

'I was in a hurry today, dashed out without breakfast and by noon I was starving. I really missed eating breakfast and noticed the difference in how I felt,' Diane remarked. When you starve during the day or your body gets attuned to not eating until the evening, you are usually famished by supper time and gobble your food down as fast as you can. Your plate is empty but do you really feel satisfied? If you skip meals you actually lower your metabolism, which is the energy required to keep your heart pumping, brain active, organs functioning, lungs breathing, and eyelids blinking. It's the level of energy needed to sustain your body's vital functions.

According to Dr Wayne Callaway's research on people who

are overweight, those who skip breakfast have metabolic rates four to five percent below normal. The meal-skipper has a mild form of starvation the same as you see in bingers. Undereating early in the day inevitably leads to overeating later on. People who snack in the evening tend to cut back the next day to make up for it. They're not hungry until they start to eat, then their appetite goes up. If they eat breakfast, they are hungry at lunch because this is part of the normal body function that has been ignored during dieting.

BREAKFAST BREAKTHROUGH

Regular eating, starting with breakfast, enhances the thermic effect of food. This can be defined as the energy expended above the resting metabolic rate for several hours after a meal. This makes you burn up more calories during and after the meal. On the other hand, extreme hunger and other factors can cause overeating in those who eat infrequently, and this may also reduce the number of calories burned because of diet-induced thermogenesis (the way individuals store and burn calories). With comparable total calories, people who eat just one meal a day have increased skinfold thicknesses (more fat), compared with those who eat more than two meals a day.[1]

Studies by Dr George Bray[2] and others have produced evidence that eating infrequent, large meals favours the storage of fat known as lipogenesis.[3] In other words, if the same number of total calories are consumed in one large meal at supper time and there is also nibbling throughout the evening, more calories will be stored as fat. Eating frequently according to your actual hunger will rev up your system. In this way you will burn more calories because of the effect of increasing the metabolic rate.

One of my clients felt famished only at the evening meal. Her system, accustomed to being without food until six o'clock, had adjusted to that time frame. When I introduced her to eating at regular times of the day, she was amazed after a period of a few weeks that she actually felt hungry at regular times. Her system adjusted to more frequent eating, and she consumed less at the evening meal.

WHY BREAKFAST?

- Try cutting back on your evening snack. Your body stores carbohydrates as glycogen, primarily in the liver. Glycogen is converted in the liver to glucose, your energy source, and released into the bloodstream as needed. These energy stores in the liver run out after about twelve hours of rest[4] (faster if you are more active, since a heavy workout can deplete your energy stores). By morning, your body will have gone about eight to twelve hours without food, and you will be ready to break the fast and refuel your energy supply.

- Traditionally, breakfast-skippers are higher on calories but shorter on nutrients, especially vitamin C which you often get from fruit or juice in the morning.

- The brain needs a steady source of glucose, the breakdown product of carbohydrates, to function. Breakfast helps to replenish this source of energy. A recent study proved that children participating in the national school breakfast programme improved more in achievement test scores than those who didn't participate. By eating breakfast you no longer need the caffeine boost to keep alert.

- Missing breakfast and starving all day, you are so hungry by dinner that you don't focus on your food or taste it, so you don't feel satisfied and may eat throughout the evening. Take the time to eat breakfast. After a few weeks, you won't be able to do without it. Taking time out for yourself will give you time back in improved productivity and you will feel better equipped to handle unexpected situations.

- During a meal it takes roughly twenty minutes for your stomach to register to your brain that you are full. If you eat too quickly it does not give you a chance to feel full. Eating regularly, including breakfast, allows you to bring more rhythm to your eating, allowing you to pace yourself and taste and enjoy the food.

- Without breakfast, your defence mechanism kicks in. Your body knows that you will feed it only once a day so it compensates by storing more of those calories as fat. It is like the squirrel who stores food for the winter. Just in case you starve yourself again, your body has something to call on.

● The brown fat that keeps the metabolic rate high is not as active if you skip breakfast because you are not eating frequently enough, which results in a lower metabolic rate. In other words, it takes calories or energy for your body to function, your heart to pump, your blood to flow, and your lungs to work.

Eating regularly involves resetting your internal clock to a regular pattern of meals. Once you begin to eat breakfast in the morning you will, within a few weeks, start to wake up hungry for the morning meal. By shifting to three regular meals a day, you will feel more energetic due to the increased effect of metabolic rate.

CARBOHYDRATES IN CONTROL

Let's work through this system of empowering you to make eating choices that make you feel satisfied for longer. Remember those foods that you often cut back on or cut out when you wanted to lose weight, those carbohydrates that you feel certain will put weight on you as soon as you eat them again? Did you ever wonder why you crave those foods? The answer is that all carbohydrates break down into sugar. If you are cutting them back, then your body makes you crave them as a defence mechanism. If you cut back on bread, cereals, potatoes, and pasta, then you will not be able to resist chocolate or a piece of cake, because your body needs sugar, natural or refined, in order to function.

Jean lamented, 'I just have to look at a piece of cake and I put on weight.' In reality, she was restricting her natural form of sugar, the carbohydrates, during the week, causing her to be in a dehydrated state due to water loss. Going out on weekends, Jean would lose control at the sweet trolley.

If you do not take in enough carbohydrates naturally, then your body will protect you by craving them from other sources, for example from cakes and biscuits. When reintroducing carbohydrates into your body, you are rehydrating yourself and therefore the immediate weight gain that follows is merely water. It is impossible to gain a couple of pounds of fat overnight.

Just as your car needs petrol to run, your body needs carbohydrates that break down into sugar to keep you going, to give you energy. Often people mistakenly believe that vitamins supply energy. Excess vitamins will not push the pace of biological reactions faster, just as having a full tank of petrol will not make a car go faster than its engine capacity will allow. Vitamins help you extract the energy from the carbohydrates, but the carbohydrates give the energy. Eating in a healthy manner provides you with a sufficient amount of vitamins and carbohydrates.

Protein is a nutrient used by the body to build and repair tissues, hormones, and enzymes. With regard to energy level, protein foods provide you with sustained energy. Foods such as meat, fish, poultry, peanut butter, eggs, and cheese give you stamina just as high octane gives mileage for the car. Protein foods allow you to extract the energy from the carbohydrates at a slower pace rather than all at once. Protein has the effect of making food 'stick to your ribs'. Eating protein foods along with carbohydrates allows the carbohydrates to break down into sugar at a slower rate, giving you more sustained energy.[5,6] Protein foods slow down the release of sugar from the carbohydrates into your bloodstream. In this way eating some protein along with carbohydrates stabilises the blood sugar swings that would otherwise lead to binges or feelings of hunger and irritability.

Fat is found hidden in protein foods as well as in recognisable fat foods such as butter, margarine, mayonnaise, or salad dressing. A certain amount of fat is needed to obtain the essential fatty acids necessary for health and wellbeing. However, these fats are the most concentrated source of calories and convert to body fat very easily. The YCCD style of living gradually cuts back on these foods through cooking tips and food choices without sacrificing flavour. It is important to make changes gradually in order to incorporate them into your lifestyle.

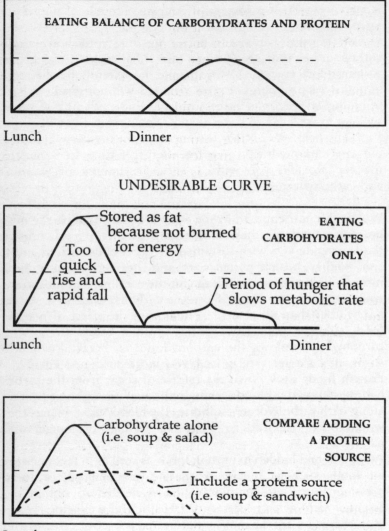

OPTIMUM CURVE

EATING BALANCE OF CARBOHYDRATES AND PROTEIN

Lunch   Dinner

UNDESIRABLE CURVE

EATING
CARBOHYDRATES
ONLY

Stored as fat
because not burned
for energy

Too
quick
rise and
rapid fall

Period of hunger that
slows metabolic rate

Lunch   Dinner

COMPARE ADDING
A PROTEIN
SOURCE

Carbohydrate alone
(i.e. soup & salad)

Include a protein source
(i.e. soup & sandwich)

Lunch   Dinner

Fat is fat, and contains the same number of calories whether it is fat from meat, margarine, butter, or oil. Vary the types of fat to decrease the total amount of saturated fat you take in. If you really like butter, do not cut it out completely. Experience has shown that people who cut butter out of their diets eventually miss it so much that they binge on it. The result is weight loss followed by a larger weight gain, and the starve/binge diet cycle rather than a new-found taste acquired from gradual changes. Attempting to cut out fat too quickly leads to only temporary change.

The principle of healthy eating is demonstrated in the chart on p106. You will find that learning to balance carbohydrate and protein choices at meals is easy. A balance is necessary at each meal to feel energetic and keep you going until the next meal. Try to watch out for fats and aim gradually to decrease the fat content of meals. Fats weigh you down and are the most concentrated source of calories, with about twice as many calories per given weight as carbohydrates and protein. Remember that high-fat foods convert to fat very efficiently. As you gradually learn to listen to your own stomach at meal times and cue in to your physical hunger needs, knowledge about the role of different food choices will then enable you to make selections that balance.

Dieters have a different attitude to food. Many are divided into 'legal' (those foods that are okay to eat when on a diet) versus 'illegal' (those foods that are the 'no-nos' of dieting).

Many dieters are not used to eating carbohydrates. They are not aware that by taking in more protein sources that contain hidden fat, they are actually 'hanging on' to fat and 'letting go' of water, along with the carbohydrate restriction. This is one of the main reasons why diets do not last. Our concept is a reverse of what dieters expect. YCCD shows you that you can eat in a healthy manner and lose body fat, not water. So learn from those former diet experiences and see them for what they are – a ploy to lose weight quickly to deceive you into thinking the diet works. **YCCD works on inner motivation that will make you feel better both inside and out. It is for the long term.**

MATTER OF BALANCE

CARBOHYDRATES	PROTEINS
Give you energy. Aim to boost energy by gradually increasing carbohydrates.	Keep you feeling full. Aim to gradually decrease protein – the next meal is just a few hours away.

Complex Carbohydrates

Bread (wholemeal grains)	Beef (lean)
Cereals (low sugar)	Pork (lean)
Pasta	Lamb (lean)
Potatoes	Chicken & Turkey
Rice	Fish & Seafood
Crackers	Game
Dried peas, Beans &	Eggs
Lentils	Cheese
(Add other vegetables	Peanut butter
for colour and texture)	

Simple Carbohydrates
Milk (natural sugar – lactose)
Starchy vegetables
(carrots, turnips, parsnips,
beets, peas, squash, corn)
Fruit

VEGETARIAN STYLE

Vegetarian eating is becoming more popular. With the emphasis on increasing carbohydrates and fibre and gradually decreasing fat content, vegetable proteins such as pulses offer those options. The function of protein with regard to health is that new protein is needed daily to allow a constant renewal of body cells and regulators, as well as to repair any damaged tissue. It's a fact that the average person in our meat-eating society takes in about twice as much protein as their body needs. This excess protein increases the overall fat content of your food intake and if it is above your energy needs for the day, it gets stored as fat.

If you eat more calories than your body needs, the excess gets stored as fat. High-fat foods, such as the hidden fat in protein foods, gets stored into fat more efficiently than high-carbohydrate foods that contain little fat.

Not all proteins are used equally by the body. The protein found in foods is not 'ready-made' to be incorporated into body tissues. Instead, the body must break it down by digestion into individual amino acids, in order to build the proteins it needs.

Although there are over twenty amino acids, only nine are essential for adults. These nine cannot be made by the body, and therefore, must be available from food sources. Proteins from animal sources such as meat, fish, poultry, eggs, milk, and milk products contain the nine essential amino acids in the proportions needed by the body. They are called 'complete' proteins. On the other hand, vegetable sources of protein are termed 'incomplete' and cannot be part of the building process unless they are combined with foods that contain the missing amino acids.

For example, pulses such as soya beans contain the highest concentration of protein in the plant world but cannot be utilised by the body unless combined with either nuts and seeds, grains, or a complete protein. You don't have to combine complementary foods at the same meal to get the effects of a complete protein. If you eat a wide variety of foods, especially if you eat even a small amount of meat or dairy products, you'll absorb a full complement of amino acids on any given day.[7] From the available data, it is reasonable to conclude that protein adequacy can be achieved when different plant proteins are eaten at separate meals throughout the course of the day.[8]

To simplify these concepts and gradually incorporate more sources of vegetable protein into your eating pattern, here are a few tips:

- *Introduce vegetable protein gradually to make it a lifestyle change and to reduce the incidence of stomach distress due to the high-fibre content.* One of my clients was used to living on salads alone (lettuce is low in fibre). When she abruptly added more grains and carbohydrates to her meals, her system became plugged. It is crucial to increase your fibre content gradually so your system can adjust.
  Note By increasing your intake of carbohydrates, you are automatically increasing the fibre content of your meals.

- *Dried beans and peas must be soaked before cooking because their skins are impermeable; water can only enter through the small end formerly attached to the plant.* (Split peas and lentils do not require pre-soaking.) To prevent gas in your stomach, soak pulses for up to five hours or overnight. Drain, add fresh water, cook for half an hour, discard water. Add more water, cook until tender and discard water a third time. The more often you change the water, the more you will reduce the gas-producing qualities of the beans. You may be getting rid of some of the water-soluble vitamin contents of the beans and some of the protein value but more importantly, you are getting rid of the component that is responsible for making you feel bloated. Adding a pinch of ginger may also help. Eat a small amount at a time until your system gets used to the fibre. In this way beans can be enjoyed for their wholesome flavour and nutrition without having any uncomfortable after-effects.

● *Drink plenty of fluids so that the fibre can allow increased movement of the intestine, thereby improving regularity and bowel movements.* Fibre acts like a sponge soaking up water. If there is not enough water around, constipation instead of regularity may result.

● *Continue to eat eggs and dairy foods.* B12 and D are found only in animal products. Plants do not contain vitamin B12. If the above foods are not eaten, soya milk or soya products fortified with vitamin B12 could be consumed.

● *A bonus of introducing more pulses to your meals is that your grocery bill will go down.* Beans, peas, and lentils are a cheap source of protein. If you don't normally use them, gradually add them to sauces and soups that you enjoy. *Tailoring Your Tastes*, our new cookbook, contains excellent ideas to incorporate pulses into your meals.

● *Meat is a good source of iron.* If plant sources of iron which include pulses, whole or enriched grains, green leafy vegetables, and other vegetables and dried fruits are used, high sources of vitamin C can be used to make more of the iron available to the body. Foods rich in vitamin C include berries, citrus fruits, tomatoes, and broccoli and could be eaten with the meal to enhance the absorption of iron.

FOOD SOURCES OF VITAMIN C

Food	Portion	Vitamin C (mg)
Orange juice (fresh)	1 cup (250 ml)	130
Grapefruit juice (fresh)	1 cup (250 ml)	94
Papayas	1/2 medium	94
Strawberries (sliced)	1 cup (250 ml)	85
Kiwi fruit	1 medium	75
Oranges	1 medium	70
Green peppers (raw)	1 medium	94
Mangoes	1 medium	57
Cantaloupe	1/4 medium	56
Cranberry juice cocktail	1/2 cup (125 ml)	54
Brussels sprouts (cooked)	4 sprouts	70
Tomato juice	1 cup (250 ml)	45
Grapefruit (white)	1/2 medium	44
Broccoli (cooked, chopped)	1/2 cup (125 ml)	75
Kale (raw, chopped)	1/2 cup (125 ml)	41
Cauliflower (raw, chopped)	1/2 cup (125 ml)	43
Potato (baked)	1 medium	26
Tangerine	1 medium	26
Tomato (raw)	1 medium	34
Cabbage (raw, shredded)	1/2 cup (125 ml)	22

If plant foods are your main source of iron, known as non-heme iron (heme iron comes from animal-derived foods), then it is crucial that you do not drink tea with your meals. If you do, iron absorption, especially non-heme iron, decreases by sixty-two percent.[9] More about this in Chapter 11 on fluids.

A vegetarian meal, such as lentil soup with bread, will fill you up sooner but will allow you to become hungry sooner. Because of the higher fibre and lower fat content of vegetable proteins when compared to animal proteins, it is normal to be hungry more quickly. As long as you understand that you may be eating more frequently throughout the day, this method of eating is an extremely healthy one.

Try using this concept of balance in your meals to give you more energy and hold you over to the next meal. If you feel hungry between meals, have a snack, otherwise overeating may occur at the next meal.

If you use pulses as your protein source, the previous chart, 'Matter of Balance', on p106 is modified.

CARBOHYDRATES	PROTEINS
Grains:	Eggs
wheat (bread, bulgar)	Cheese
Rice	Milk
Corn	Peanut butter
Oats	Pulses:
Pasta	dried peas
Cereal	(yellow or green peas,
Potatoes	chick peas,
Fruit†	black-eye peas)
Vegetables†	Dry beans:
	kidney beans,
	soya beans
	Nuts*
	Seeds*

† Simple carbohydrates such as fruits and vegetables can be added to meals for the feeling of fullness and the vitamins and minerals they offer. However, except for corn, these foods cannot be used to make a protein complete and usable by the body.
* Nuts and seeds are both high in carbohydrate and incomplete as vegetable protein and are also high in fat content. Use them sparingly.

● *Focus on gradually increasing the carbohydrate content of your meals, but include enough protein to keep you feeling satisfied.* Note that due to the lower fat content of vegetable protein foods, you may feel hungry sooner than if you ate a balanced meal that included animal protein. The reason for this is that animal protein contains hidden fat that adds to the feeling of fullness. Remember, carbohydrates digest more quickly, giving you an immediate energy boost. Protein foods take longer to digest and keep you feeling satisfied longer. A balanced meal will probably be sufficient for three to six hours, depending on fat content.

Allow this period of time between meals and actually experience physical hunger. Constant eating will not allow you this experience. But do not go to extremes. Eating only three meals a day could leave you famished by mealtime, decreasing your opportunity to taste and savour your food.

I usually experience a dual reaction in my class when participants are told that they can have any food they want, including
the conventional 'forbidden when dieting' list. People exhibit a
sense of relief along with a sense of fear. A possible consequence
without the new perspective is that a continued sense of
restriction may cause them to overeat until they gain the
confidence from their developing control over food. For some
people, keeping a journal of what they eat (no quantities) and
how they feel will help them on the process of self-discovery.

Deprivation that occurred due to previous attempts to diet
leads to a rebellion causing overeating. If this is happening to
you, become aware of why it is happening and focus on tuning
into your true physical hunger, using the eating guidelines to
reduce the number of urges that may occur. Eating more
carbohydrates and obtaining natural sugar from them will
decrease your urge for sweets. These foods will provide you
with your energy source. Giving yourself permission to eat what
you want and not following a structured diet does not mean that
there is no focus. Trust yourself to find your balance and beware
of your pendulum swinging the other way.

Check your balance at each meal using the form provided on
p112 to indicate the types of food you are eating. If you would
like to check out your understanding of the principles of healthy
eating, an individual assessment of your journal can be done to
determine to what extent your eating habits are in balance. (See
order form at end of book for details.)

Many of our present eating habits are in the form of
a triangle, that is we eat less during the day and more in the
evening. Try to gradually reverse this order. Start with a more
hearty breakfast, a more substantial lunch, and even though
your evening meal may be large, it probably will be less than you
used to eat. Any weight gain that may occur may be due to one
of the following reasons:

- Rehydration of water stores with reintroduction of carbohydrates because carbohydrates are stored with water. This is
'water' weight, not 'fat' weight.

- Overeating due to 'permission to eat'.

- Not yet tuned into your natural hunger signals (more about
this in Chapter 6).

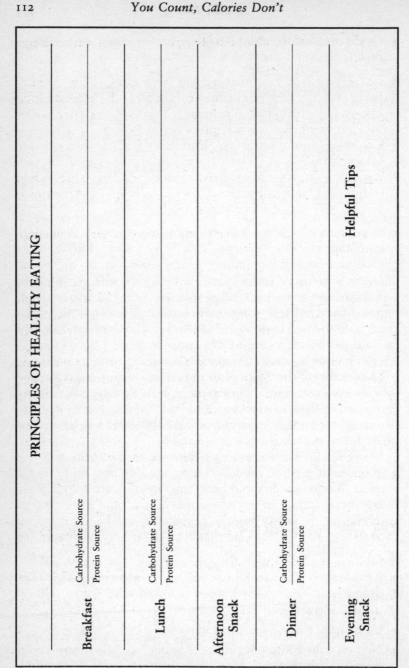

PRINCIPLES OF HEALTHY EATING

Breakfast
Carbohydrate Source
Protein Source

Lunch
Carbohydrate Source
Protein Source

Afternoon Snack

Dinner
Carbohydrate Source
Protein Source

Evening Snack

Helpful Tips

- Overeating as a result of rebellion to dieting (starvation/binge cycle).

- Overeating since increasing carbohydrates. This implies being 'off the diet' and time to binge on those foods long known to be forbidden (i.e. bread). You need to switch out of the diet mentality (see Chapters 6 and 7).

- Retaining water due to insufficient fluid intake (see Chapter 11).

- Retaining fluid due to excessive consumption of foods high in sodium (i.e. salt, convenience foods, carbonated diet drinks, pickles, soy sauce, some snack foods).

- Increase in muscle mass due to increase in activity. A positive outcome!

I used to skip breakfast and eat very little, if anything, at lunch. This led to a huge supper, and people were amazed at how much I could devour. Then in my mid twenties the weight began to catch up with me. I realised that this style of eating eventually catches up with even naturally slip people. It takes longer in men due to their greater muscle mass as a result of body composition.

The first step is to learn how to satisfy your physical hunger by balancing your meals with carbohydrate and protein content that best suit your needs. You don't have to purchase a new set of cookbooks or recipe books or spend a lot of time preparing meals by following elaborate time-consuming recipes. Simply fine-tune your present eating habits to ensure that you are eating in a balanced way.

GETTING THE MOST ENERGY OUT OF FOODS

Here are some examples of meals with the right balance.

Breakfast
Natural Jump-starters:

Carbohydrate bread, muffins, fruit, crackers, pancakes, cereal, potatoes, milk, bagels.

Many store-bought or restaurant muffins may be high in fat

content and contain up to 400–500 calories (see Chapters 5 and 10). However, fat is being purged from some commercial muffins as consumers become more health conscious. Croissants may sound light and airy, but they contain twice the fat of a biscuit and six times the fat of an English muffin.

Protein   cheese, peanut butter, eggs, meat, grilled bacon.

Try toast with low-fat cheese melted on top (no butter or margarine since there is hidden fat in the cheese). To make it even more special, put onions, tomatoes, courgette, pepper, or any other vegetable on the toast before adding the cheese. Also great for lunch!

Try peanut butter and jam or banana on toast! If you have frozen raspberries on hand, pop in the microwave just until defrosted and spread on top of the peanut butter for a new taste sensation that is sure to be a hit!

Note   No butter or margarine is needed since there is hidden fat in peanut butter.

Try poached, scrambled, or fried egg (with a little fat) on toast. Or try toast with quark, or ricotta cheese with jam, canned fruit (preserved in its own juice), or fresh fruit cut up on top.

Note   Quark is a low-fat cheese that tastes similar to cream cheese. However, it is very bland in flavour and therefore the jam adds just the right flavour stimulation. Try wholemeal toast with quark and cut up strawberries. If the strawberries are frozen, pop them in the microwave just until defrosted but still firm. This is refreshing and appealing! There are also a variety of other low-fat spreadable cheese products on the market that are full of flavour. Of course, cottage cheese is one of the cheeses lowest in fat content. The above cheeses provide variety and alternatives for those who leave cottage cheese to go mouldy in the refrigerator.

Try pancakes and cheese. Incorporate your favourite type of fruit into the pancake mix for added moisture. When serving, spread quark on top instead of syrup for some protein source at this meal. Tastes rich.

Add cereal and milk, fruit, or greater quantities of food to the food list to give you a feeling of satisfaction, without being overly full. The examples given will help you to understand the balance.

Lunch

Gradually increase the carbohydrate content of your meals and gradually decrease your protein content so that you have energy and feel satisfied for a longer period of time. The word 'gradual' is emphasised, because human nature tends to make you want everything to happen immediately. Focus on lifestyle change, not the diet mentality.

Note If you have been restricting carbohydrates in the past, it is normal to gain three to four pounds (one to two kg) to replenish your carbohydrate stores. The body has to store carbohydrates with water. It takes three to four pounds (one to two kg) of water to store one pound (0.5 kg) of glycogen (stored form of carbohydrates). When people begin to reintroduce carbohydrates into their way of eating, they often feel bloated. They do not recognise this sensation as a normal result of eating sufficient carbohydrates.

Carbohydrate   bread, bagels, pita bread, fruit, pasta, potatoes, rice, milk, yogurt, vegetables.

Note Vegetables that you pull from the ground such as carrots, parsnips, beets, and turnips as well as corn, squash, and peas are the starchy ones. The other vegetables can be used as a filler. They contain vitamins and minerals, and are not considered part of the carbohydrate component of the meal due to high water content with very little carbohydrate content. Include both complex and simple carbohydrates at each meal (refer to 'Matter of Balance' for examples, p106).

Protein   leftover meat, canned fish, eggs, peanut butter, cheese, pulses (peas, beans, lentils), milk, yogurt. Gradually try some of the low-fat cheeses.

Sandwiches are great quick lunches. Sometimes people don't care for bread because they haven't given themselves a chance to experiment with the wide variety of tastes and flavours available today. You may like breads that are coarser (wholemeal or any form of whole grain). However, beware of bread that contains

caramel colouring and has a soft texture. Read the label. This
bread is probably not whole grain.

Fillers in sandwiches can be anything. Try leftover chicken,
beef, pork, canned tuna, salmon, or other canned fish, cheese,
peanut butter, or egg. Luncheon meats are used less frequently
because of higher fat content. If using canned fish, try to
purchase it packed in water or, if packed in oil, rinse and
use less fat to moisten the sandwich. If you use a light
mayonnaise mixed with the canned fish, adding butter or
margarine to the bread as well is not necessary.

Retrain your taste buds. Consider making toast. You take a
piece of bread, toast it, and in this way get rid of the moisture in
exchange for texture. Then you add butter or margarine to
bring back the moisture and get rid of the texture. Does this
make sense? Focus your taste on the texture and flavour rather
than the greasy mushy taste. Often when margarine is cut back
or even eliminated on toast and replaced with a protein food
such as cheese or peanut butter that contains hidden fat, the
butter or margarine is not missed. Was it more a habit than a
desire? Changing the habit does not instil feelings of deprivation. Focus on progress and lifestyle adjustments rather than
immediate temporary change.

Remember that weight is not necessarily an indicator of health.
Alice, a client in her twenties, was referred to me for weight
counselling. She weighed 311 pounds (141 kg) and had not been
on many previous diets. Every time she even thought about
going on a diet, she would crave food and binge, so the diets
were short-lived. But she was receptive to trying a lifestyle
approach where the focus of success would be improved
health. Months later, Alice made a number of remarkable
changes: she reduced by half the number of times she had to
take ventolin for her asthma, she ate differently because she
wanted to, her food tasted better, and she prepared food that
had a low-fat content. She began to walk regularly and enjoyed
it. Her clothes were a little looser even though her weight was
down only slightly. The physical improvement was gradual, not
instant.

Alice was much healthier, but by society's measure of success,
which is weight, she had failed. Focusing on weight, conven-

tional counsellors might have advised Alice to decrease her food intake and increase her activity. She would have been required to work above her comfort zone. This may have had a negative effect on her health.

When Alice followed my advice to focus on her lifestyle adjustments, this created the momentum to continue with the plan. Her focus was entirely off weight. She accepted that it would take two to five years to internalise the lifestyle changes, but she was enjoying the process so time wasn't an issue.

Since both of Alice's parents were large, Alice had an eighty percent change of being large as well. With lifestyle changes in place her body will naturally adjust to the weight it is genetically meant to be. Society's expectations that all women should be within a certain range of weights is not the issue here. It is a woman's long-term health that is important. Alice did not fail. She enjoyed striving to be the best that she could be!

Dieters are used to skimping on bread and making open sandwiches using the thinly sliced bread available in supermarkets. But you can be much more satisfied by eating more bread without guilt. If you allow yourself to feel guilty while consuming more carbohydrates, then you are not allowing yourself to experience the excitement of tasting and savouring your food. This will result in eating more food in order to feel satisfied.

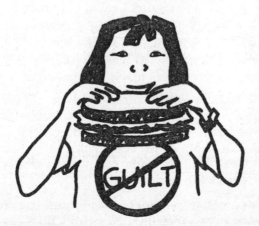

Making sandwiches with thicker slices of bread makes you feel as if you have something in your hand. It can be very satisfying. Cut thick slices of bread and put enough filler to keep you satisfied, or have two sandwiches. It is not the quantity that counts, it is the balance in eating and the total fat content that will make the difference. Try adding mustard, light salad dressing, or tomato and lettuce to sandwiches instead of always using butter or margarine.

Add soup or salad if you like. Try varying types of bread or using pita pockets. Another option that is quick for lunch is a stir-fry made with leftovers from the fridge. Use a teflon frying pan and a cover to contain moisture which will reduce the total fat content needed. Leftover chicken, beef, potatoes, rice, and vegetables work well. If the mixture starts to stick, add a little liquid such as water, water with a stock cube, juice, or leftover low-fat gravy.

Soups can be made hearty by adding a protein source such as cheese, leftover meat, chicken, pulses such as lentils, beans, and a carbohydrate source such as potatoes, rice, or barley. Eat the soup with some bread or rolls. If the soup is not substantial enough, you will probably be hungry a couple of hours later. Experiment and learn the quantity that you need.

Snacks

Some form of complex carbohydrate such as bread, rolls, crackers, cold pizza, bulgur, lentils, or fruit alone, cheese with fruit, popcorn (watch the butter), milk, or yogurt is good for a snack. Milk and yogurt contain some protein as well and therefore may serve as a more satisfying snack. Milk products also ensure that you get enough calcium during the day.

Supper

Most people tend to eat balanced meals at supper but they usually emphasise the protein source. Try to ensure that you are increasing your carbohydrate source and gradually decreasing your protein source, but do eat enough protein to hold you over till the next meal. Find the right balance of carbohydrate and protein that works for you.

Carbohydrate pasta, potatoes, rice, bread, crackers, fruit, milk, yogurt, starchy vegetables. *Note* Milk does contain some protein but it is also very high in carbohydrate. Due to its liquid form and the fact that it is relatively low in protein, it is not very satisfying and has little 'holding over' power. For this reason, it is found under the carbohydrate section.

Protein   lean beef, lean pork, lean lamb, lean chicken, turkey, fish, liver, game, eggs, cheese, pulses, peanut butter.

Do not eat only chicken and fish. Beef and pork are much leaner than they used to be (see Chapter 5). Where does portion control or measuring your three ounces (eighty-five grams) of meat fit into all this you ask? Rather than becoming preoccupied with quantities, aim for balance.

● As a check for a healthy balance learn to observe what's on your plate. Aim for two-thirds to three-quarters carbohydrates and one-third to one-quarter protein content. Learn to recognise the balance that is right for you rather than measuring how much you need. This balance will give you energy and keep you going.

● Tune into your internal signals of hunger and fullness for quantities that you need to satisfy you.

Remember that counting exchanges leaves you preoccupied with food and does not allow you the opportunity to work with your body. Getting back in touch with your body will give you the confidence to listen to it for the quantities you need to maintain energy and health.

COOKING FOR ONE OR TWO

Make a larger roast or cook greater quantities of food (more pork chops, larger chicken, more hamburgers, large bean casserole) plus more rice, potatoes, or pasta. Divide meat into freezer containers, cool, add gravy (use ice cube tip as explained in Chapter 5), package, and put in the freezer for those rushed days or those 'I don't feel like cooking' days.

Note Pasta and rice will freeze but potatoes do not freeze well. Reheat leftovers for breakfast or lunch. Add vegetables or a salad.

Note Meat and carbohydrates (pasta and rice) keep for a few days in the fridge. Freezing them just gives you more variety, the easy way.

CARBOHYDRATES FOR THE MOST ENERGY

Even if you don't like vegetables you can acquire a taste for them if you introduce them gradually.

Balance and variety are important to gradually introduce more vegetables as you experiment with foods. A way of eating that is rich in fruits, vegetables, and grains may protect you against many kinds of disorders including cancer. Promising research suggests that the so-called antioxidant nutrients such as beta carotene (which the body converts into vitamin A), vitamin C, and other substances in fruits and vegetables may help ward off certain cancers.

When John started the programme, he didn't like vegetables. In balancing carbohydrates and proteins, he would choose more grains than fruits and vegetables. Then gradually, without being forced to, he acquired a taste for some of these other foods. By the end of the programme, he was discovering the new taste sensations of vegetables for himself.

Try the darker green leaf lettuce. The darker the leaves, the more nutritious. For example, romaine lettuce has about six times as much vitamin C and eight times as much beta carotene as iceberg lettuce.[10] Be adventurous. Eat 'cooking greens' raw sometimes and salad greens cooked.

Normally if you eat only carbohydrates at a meal, you will feel hungry very soon since carbohydrates are digested and absorbed into your bloodstream quickly. But what about snacks? Carbohydrate foods make ideal snacks where the purpose is simply to keep ou going to the next meal. However, carbohydrates alone can cause an immediate rise then fall in blood sugar. This effect of low blood sugar will make you feel tired and hungry again. To prevent this, choose carbohydrates that give you a more gradual rise in blood sugar and are therefore more effective in holding you over till the next meal.

The complex carbohydrates (breads, pasta, potatoes, rice, pulses) consist of a longer chain molecule. Chemically, they take longer to break down than the simple carbohydrates (milk, vegetables, fruit, sugar, honey). Using this theory you should focus on consuming more complex carbohydrate foods.

The entire focus up to this point has been to increase the quantity of carbohydrates that you may be consuming. This has been done by including a variety of both complex and simple carbohydrates. With meals, a source of protein has been included to provide a better balance. In the process you may have discovered that certain carbohydrate foods are more effective than others in keeping you satisfied at snack time. Why is this?

Tests have been done using different carbohydrate foods to discover how these foods would affect blood sugar physiologically. Individuals ingested one-ounce (28-g) portions of carbohydrate foods and were tested to see the effect this had on blood sugar levels. A glycaemic index table was the result. This table provides a method of rating selected carbohydrate-rich foods according to how high they elevate blood sugar levels. The higher the glycaemic index, the more the food elevates blood glucose levels, thereby releasing glucose (sugar) more quickly into the bloodstream. The glycaemic index indicates that your blood sugar will shoot up faster following a snack of potatoes, carrots, or bread, than after a snack of fruit, pulses (beans, peas, or lentils), nuts, or pasta.

Some high-fibre foods can keep blood glucose from soaring after a meal by releasing glucose, our form of energy, in small doses. This prevents blood sugar from going on a roller coaster ride that will cause energy levels to dip. High-fibre foods achieve this by delaying food release from the stomach, and by slowing the digestion of starch and sugars in the intestine. With a slower release of glucose into the bloodstream (flatter glucose response), you have a more sustained energy level.

Other factors that affect glycaemic response are:

● the amount and type of fibre;

● the form the food is in (i.e. the smoother the texture, the higher the glycaemic response);

● the degree to which the food is cooked;

- the speed of eating; and
- timing the consumption of liquids.

FASTER ←─────────────────────────────────

THE GLYCAEMIC INDEX[11]
(rated from quickest glucose release to slowest)

baked potato (russet)	brown rice	orange juice
honey	raisins	whole grain rye bread
corn flakes	wheat crackers	apples
instant potatoes	sucrose (table sugar)	dairy products
millet	frozen peas	beans/pulses
white/wholemeal bread	porridge-style oatmeal	plums
corn	banana	cherries
Mars Bar	buckwheat	fructose (fruit sugar)
white rice	sweet potato	peanuts
	pasta	
	oranges	

─────────────────────────────────→ SLOWER

THE 'HOW MUCH' AND 'HOW-TO' OF FIBRE

We used to hear a lot about wheat bran. Lately the emphasis has switched to oat bran and its effect on cholesterol. There is no need for confusion – both of these foods contain fibre. However, the type of fibre and its function are different. Water-insoluble fibres, such as wheat bran, can improve bowel regularity. Water-soluble fibres become gel-like during digestion; they are the ones that seem to help keep blood glucose and cholesterol levels in line. Ensure a gradual increase in fibre content to minimise stomach distress, bloating, and discomfort as well as the focus on lifestyle change. Drink plenty of fluids, especially with insoluble fibre so that it will be able to perform its function of regularity.

Fructose is a major carbohydrate component of fruits. It takes much longer to release glucose into your system than table sugar (sucrose) because the body must first convert it to glucose before it can be used or stored. In particular, fruits and vegetables high in natural pectin are lower on the glycaemic index.

SOURCES OF DIETARY FIBRE

SOLUBLE *High in pectins and gums*	INSOLUBLE *High in cellulose,* *hemicelluloses, and lignin*
dried peas, beans, lentils	bran cereals
seeds	whole grain cereals
nuts	whole grain breads & rolls
raw fruits	whole grain crackers
dried fruits	whole grains
raw vegetables	brown rice
cooked vegetables	cracked wheat
oat bran	bulgur

Pectin is a gel-like substance that delays emptying of the stomach. In this way, it makes you feel fuller longer, causing a slower release of glucose into the bloodstream. Fruits and vegetables high in pectin are high in soluble fibre. Fruits and vegetables high in pectin are squash, apples, cauliflower, citrus fruits (grapefruits, oranges), green beans, cabbage, carrots, strawberries, potatoes, dried peas.

Dried fruit may be high in soluble fibre but it also contains a concentrated sugar source because the moisture has been taken out. Fresh fruit or fruit canned in its own juice would be a more refreshing choice that would satisfy both hunger and thirst. Even though nuts and seeds are high in soluble fibre and contain some vegetable protein, they are also high in hidden fat. It is easy to eat a cup (250 ml) of peanuts at once without even realising it. However, along with the peanuts go 900 calories of which 684 calories come from fat. Why did you eat them? Much of this eating may even be unconscious eating where you are not even tasting the food. A more satisfying choice at roughly 170 total calories would be a slice of bread with a tablespoon (fifteen mL) of peanut butter. By adding the carbohydrate source, the total fat content is essentially reduced and a better balance exists. Only eighty-one calories, or forty-seven percent of the calories, come from fat as opposed to seventy-six percent of the calories coming from fat by eating the peanuts alone.

Increasing soluble-fibre contents such as fruits, vegetables, and oat bran causes a total decrease in the amount of saturated fat in your total eating pattern. Saturated fat is often used in convenience foods in the form of hydrogenated vegetable oil to improve the shelf life of the product. It has the effect of elevating cholesterol levels. However, soluble fibre forms a gel-like substance as it is digested, and it stays in your stomach longer, keeping you full for a longer period of time. It is for this reason that a breakfast consisting of oatmeal porridge may be just as satisfying as a breakfast containing a protein source. You can add fruit and some milk to the porridge to add more fibre as well as a little protein.

Oat bran does not have any flavour of its own and dissolves in liquids. To help incorporate more fibre into your meals, try adding oat bran to the following dishes:

- in hamburgers as a binder instead of crackers or bread crumbs (wheat bran can also be used);
- in muffins;
- in spaghetti meat sauce, stews, or soups as a thickener;
- as toppings on canned fruit, yogurt, or puddings;
- in chili and meat loaf; and
- in batters for pancakes, waffles, and Yorkshire puddings.

FOOD FORM

The form the food is in has a bearing on how effective it will be in satisfying you. Insoluble fibre such as that found in whole grain products adds texture to food. Since it needs to be chewed more and takes longer to eat, it helps to extend the meal. Pasta is lower on the glycaemic index indicating that the sugar is released more slowly into the bloodstream. The compact nature of the starch in pasta reduces accessibility of the starch to digestive enzymes that are involved in breaking down the starch molecule. It takes longer for the starch molecule to break down into sugar and this causes the slower release of the sugar into the bloodstream.

Whole grain rather than wholemeal products result in flatter glucose responses keeping you satisfied longer. You can achieve this by:

- parboiling wheat to form bulgur;
- parboiling rice to reduce the gelatinisation of the starch (the bonus is that this parboiled rice, known as converted rice, involves a process by which the nutrients are pushed back into the grain resulting in a greater retention of minerals and vitamins in the cooked grain); and
- use of whole cereal grain in pumpernickel bread, a whole grain rye bread.

Note Flour made from whole wheat grains will produce brown-coloured bread. But a colouring agent could be used to make brown bread from white flour. To make sure, check the list of ingredients on the label. When brown bread is not made with whole wheat flour, that is when molasses or caramel is used to colour the bread, the words 'made without whole wheat flour' or 'coloured with . . .' must appear on the label according to law.[13] Read your labels!

Note Potatoes have a greater response on blood sugar levels than rice, spaghetti, or lentils because of the food form. Using whole potatoes with the skin rather than mashed potatoes can change this response. When making chipped or mashed potatoes, try leaving the skin on for the added fibre and colour.

Grinding or cooking a starchy food as in mashed potatoes speeds up the food's absorption in the intestine, causing blood glucose to rise more rapidly.

COOKING FOOD

Try to eat more raw vegetables and fruit. Cook vegetables only to the crisp stage. When foods are raw, the cellulose cell walls are not completely disrupted by chewing. These prevent the digestive enzymes reaching the starch within the cell. Cooking swells the starch within the cell, bursting the cell wall and potentially making the starch more available for digestion.

SPEED OF EATING

Eating slowly maximises your enjoyment of food and provides an earlier feeling of satiety for a given quantity of food consumed. Slow eating will slow down the release of sugar into your bloodstream. Eating quickly minimises your enjoyment of food and fools your body's defence against eating too much. Remember that it takes roughly twenty minutes for your stomach to tell your brain it's full.

TIMING CONSUMPTION OF LIQUIDS

When liquids are ingested along with solid foods, they empty more rapidly from the stomach into the small intestine. So if you are consuming liquids containing sugar, drink these fluids after a meal. Better yet, keep in diluting those liquids whether they are juices or drinks. You will end up with a beverage that is more refreshing and does wonders for quenching your thirst.

If you find a particular carbohydrate food makes you hungry when eaten alone, try adding a source of protein.

By focusing on increasing the carbohydrate content of your meals, you already have decreased the overall fat content. Ensure that you are eating a variety of sources of carbohydrates to get the benefits of regularity, satiety, and a sustained energy source. The next step will be to learn ways to gradually decrease the fat content by preparing foods tastefully with less fat.

ACTION POINTS

- Eat regularly every four to six hours beginning with breakfast. Snacks are part of regular eating to keep your body fuelled for energy.

- Eat foods you fancy and enjoy – without feeling guilty.

- Eat a balance of carbohydrates and protein that suit you, gradually increasing the balance to include more carbohydrates and less protein.

- Add more fibre to your meals a little at a time. Notice how it fills you up more quickly and gives texture to meals. To allow fibre to work properly in your body, it's important to ensure you drink enough liquids. Tailor your tastes to appreciate these new flavours and textures.

- Notice how you feel when you are:

  eating regularly;

  hungry;

  full; and

  changing the balance of carbohydrates and protein.

- Eat when you are pleasantly hungry, not starved. This will allow you to pay attention to your food and eat more slowly.

- Stop eating when you are comfortably full, not stuffed.

- Maximise your enjoyment of food by tasting and savouring it. You will end up eating more slowly.

5

Tailoring Your Tastes

Taking the focus off fat

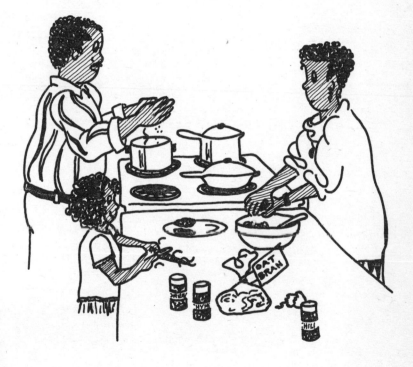

Is the obsession moving from counting grams of carbohydrate, calories, or exchanges to counting grams of fat? Is this simply a repackaging of the same old diet message, where the focus is still on numbers rather than on satiety and enjoyment of taste and texture? The answer is yes. Look round you critically and begin to evaluate the new language people are using, the talk in the staff room, the commercials on television. This is not about a new lifestyle – this is the same message repackaged to fool the consumer that the intentions of the weight-loss industry are real and valid. The fear of fat on one's body is now transferred to a fear of eating too much fat in food. Rigidly restricting fat in our food simply replaces an obsession about body fat with counting the amount of fat grams in our food, and adds to our health problems.

Take a look at how you feel about fat in the food you eat. Ask yourself these questions:

- Am I counting the number of grams of fat in the food I eat?

- Do I base decisions about what foods to eat on the amount of fat in the food?

- Am I attempting to cut out all fat in my food?

- Am I afraid of fat on my body and fat in food?

- Am I accepting society's message that this behaviour is normal and healthy?

- Does my conversation revolve around food, fat and fibre?

- Is this way of thinking making me obsessed with numbers, calories, or fat grams, and is it making me feel bad about myself?

- Am I restricting my fat intake too much, resulting in hunger, cravings, and feelings of deprivation?

- Do I binge on high-fat foods when I get the chance.

- Do I deny the need to eat some fat for my physical health and enjoyment of food?

If you answered yes to one or more of these questions, then you need to recognise that you can choose to buy into this way of thinking or make some changes.

WHY DO WE NEED TO EAT SOME FAT?

Healthwise, a small amount of fat in our daily eating pattern is needed to give us the essential fatty acids we need. Fat is also necessary to act as a carrier for fat-soluble vitamins.[1] Just as importantly, fat helps our food to taste and feel good. It makes us feel full and helps to keep us full for a longer period of time because it takes time for us to digest it.

Why the concern about fat in food? In the past, foods with a higher fat content were prized because they were not as easily found in nature. We have come a long way since then. Today convenience foods, which are generally higher in fat content than foods prepared from scratch or in their fresh form, are readily available. In recent years investigators have found evidence that the body may be able to convert dietary fat into body fat with greater ease than it can convert carbohydrates (starches and sugars) into body fat.[2–4] In other words, it takes more energy to convert carbohydrates into body fat than to convert fat calories into fat tissue.

In class, when Barbara heard this, she felt that she had to cut back her fat intake even more. She was consuming very little fat to begin with – only in cooking and on her salad. Eating too much fat is not desirable for overall health, but dieters can actually restrict their fat consumption too much. Remember those days when people used to restrict carbohydrates (those foods that contain natural sugar, like bread, potatoes and pasta) only to crave those foods later on? The same process may be occurring with fat. Denying yourself fat can lead to feelings of deprivation, increased cravings, and binging. The purpose is not to go down to the bare minimum of fat, which is the diet mentality. You might end up feeling psychologically deprived and binging on higher-fat items. Take it gradually. The taste for a lower-fat way of eating will come with time.

Today people are more conscious of their fat intake and are consuming less butter and meat. However, their total daily fat intake has not decreased. How can this be? Even though people are eating less meat, trimming the fat off the meat they do eat, and consuming less butter, their fat intake often remains high because there has been an increase in the purchase of such foods as premium ice cream, gourmet soups, and convenience foods such as processed meats. These items are high in fat. If you eat them often, you have not learned to enjoy the taste and texture of lower-fat foods. You have simply shifted the source of your fat consumption. The visible fat is being traded for the hidden fat that you don't actually see.

WHERE DOES MEAT FIT IN?

Eating more grains, pulses, fruits, and vegetables instead of convenience foods and protein foods, such as processed meats, gives better health and the bonus of a reduced grocery bill. However, some people have cut down on beef and pork and are eating more fish and poultry in the belief that these items are leaner. Not so, because modern meat sources contain less fat than animals raised years ago.[5] In fact, beef steak has the same fat content as the white meat of chicken breast with the skin removed.

Note The type of fish and preparation method will determine whether the fish has a high fat content. Vary the types of fish you eat since fish such as salmon, herring, sardines, mackerel, tuna, and trout contain a higher amount of omega-3 fatty acids, which seem to have the effect of lowering blood cholesterol levels.

Ann would not eat pork and beef because she thought they were too high in fat. But her lunches would often consist of deep-fried chicken or burgers, garlic toast, and chips. All these items are high in fat, and Ann added even more fat by topping them with greasy gravy. Was she compensating for the fact that she liked fat and was cutting it out too quickly by eliminating pork and beef? Adding gravy to chips did not allow her to tune into the crispness (texture) of the chips. The idea is not to eat one way at home, 'being good all week', only to binge on high-fat foods when you go out, or on weekends, as 'your reward'. You are not dieting – you are developing a new lifestyle where your new-found preferences help you to make healthier choices more frequently.[6]

In another situation, Donna decided to use margarine instead of butter as she enjoyed the taste of butter but did not care for margarine. Her thinking was that if she didn't like margarine she would not eat as much of it and would therefore decrease the amount of fat she was taking in. This is in fact what happened in the short term. She did eat less margarine and therefore less total fat, but a few months later her craving for butter became so strong that she ended up binging on the butter. Sudden decreases in fat content are recognised as being part of the dieting process. Attempts to restrict higher-fat foods while people still have a preference for these foods result in feelings of deprivation and may cause a higher intake of fat than would normally be consumed.[7]

The starve/binge cycle that occurs with sweets is now also occurring with fats. Part of the reason for this increase is the tendency to make changes in one's eating patterns too quickly. Sudden changes may turn out to be only temporary changes. Compare the big jump to the smooth slide in the chart on p135 and decide for yourself which you prefer.

Jane, who is a long-time dieter, ate cottage cheese and fruit every time she was on a diet. The problem was that she did not like the taste or texture of cottage cheese so her new way of eating did not become a lifestyle change. It was only something temporary that she did in order to lose weight. Resuming old habits of eating once the weight has been lost leads to weight gain. And then the cycle brings you right back to the same ineffective and unappetising eating habits in order to lose weight. To succeed, break the diet cycle.

The best plan is to fine-tune your present eating habits. Start from where you are right now and implement gradual changes to allow your entire household to acquire a taste for a healthier way of eating. Begin by ensuring that you have a balanced menu and then gradually make changes to bring out new flavours and textures.

The BIG Decision
Moving to healthier eating.

	THE BIG JUMP	THE SMOOTH SLIDE
First action on decision	BRACE YOURSELF. Quickly eat all of your favourite foods because they won't be part of your diet tomorrow.	LOOK AT YOURSELF & FEEL GOOD ABOUT YOU! Feel good that you have made the conscious decision to start making slow changes that will reflect a healthier lifestyle.
First shopping trip for healthy food	Stock up on foods that are 'light', 'low-fat' and/or 'diet' on the labels regardless of whether you enjoy them. Your household like whole milk but now that you've made the decision to 'go healthy', you buy skimmed milk.	Stock up on a wide variety of foods that you and your household enjoy, paying more attention to moving towards more carbohydrate foods and less protein. Buy a few herbs to highlight the flavours of your foods. Your family likes whole milk, so now you buy some semi-skimmed milk and plan to serve it to your family. If they don't like it at first, you can mix it half & half with whole milk till they prefer the lighter taste.
Feelings of cook after one week	Frustrated & overwhelmed. Food is drier than the family enjoys. Still has strong resolve to keep this up, even if rest of family isn't as enthusiastic.	Encouraged by how easy it has been to make small changes to the foods, cooking techniques and carbohydrate/protein balance that they already enjoy. Surprised that no one has complained or even really noticed the changes. Notices that the foods have a nicer colour and texture with all the taste they had before.
Reaction of family after one week	Concerned that the food will never be 'tasty' any more. Tired of the new chewier, drier tastes & textures of these new foods. Longing for last week's menu. Quite agile at slipping food to grateful canine under – table. Wishing that the budget allowed more take aways for next week. Snacking and eating away from home as much as possible.	Surprised that even though the decision to 'go healthy' was made, they still get to eat the foods they love! Noticed that the foods they loved have more colour and just as much, if not more, flavour than before. Feel more energised after they eat rather than tired and overfull.
Feelings of cook at one month	Almost ready to give up because no one (including the cook) is enjoying the food that is prepared. Disappointed & feeling deprived. Misses cooking and eating all the foods that they used to eat. Wishes that cooking wouldn't be such an overwhelming chore. Sneaking 'favourites' more and more often.	Excited that the process is still so enjoyable; not even thinking about giving up; having more and more fun experimenting with old and new recipes; pleased with the results, flavours, and textures.
Reaction of family at one month	Ready to move to the neighbours during meal times. Wishing the 'health kick' that hit the house would stop kicking. Eating out or having take aways as much as possible and, when eating foods they enjoy, really eating lots. Snacking and sneaking foods that they love on a more and more frequent basis.	Still enjoying the food that is on the table. Asking for certain favourites more often, 'When are you going to make that great bread again?' Noticing that they aren't hungry between meals as often.
Situation at three months	Disillusioned with the 'health movement'. Feeling disappointed and a little guilty, they give up and return to the old ways of eating and cooking again. Some of the family feels only 'joy' because they finally get to eat what they love!	Feel good about themselves and their new ways of eating and preparing foods. Energised by the successes, the whole household wants to keep moving on the smooth side towards healthier eating. As an experiment, they try some of the old ways of cooking and eating. They are surprised and pleased to find that they actually like the new ways better. They prefer the new flavours, textures and tastes and don't want to go back.

© 1995 Adapted from *Tailoring Your Tastes* by Linda Omichinski, RD & Heather Wiebe Hildebrand, RN.

BALANCE IN LIFE: Healthy Living

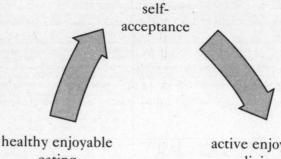

self-
acceptance

healthy enjoyable
eating

active enjoyable
living

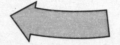

Many people are enthusiastic about a new way of eating at the beginning of the programme but they give up because trying new ideas seems too much trouble. This process is actually easier than switching to new recipes and foods. You don't have to spend time gathering new recipes and buying new ingredients to get on the road to healthier eating. When you try to alter your recipes drastically, then you are switching back into the diet mentality. It is better to adjust your present recipes while retaining, even enhancing, the flavour and texture you are used to. Otherwise, you may bake and eat flavourless cakes that do not satisfy you, and this inevitably leads to binging on the cakes you do like. When you are out of the diet mentality, you will eat only one or two biscuits at a time instead of six or the whole packet of biscuits. Making a diet recipe that contains half the calories and eating twice as much is not the way to change your tastes and listen to your body.

Putting the YCCD philosophy into practice by gradually cutting back fat content does not mean eliminating fat. Otherwise you will miss the flavours you enjoy, feel deprived, and become very discouraged.

Sylvia had a hard time accepting the idea of gradual change.

'But I have a friend who eats in a healthy way and exercises regularly and she looks great. So why can't I do it too?' She wanted immediate results. I eventually discovered that Sylvia's friend puts all her efforts into looking good and doing things just right. Then she gets fed up and reverts to her old behaviour. Apparently she does this several times throughout the year. If you constantly compare yourself to others, you will be wasting your energy on wishful thinking rather than action. Remember, you are doing this for yourself for your lifetime. Do it gradually, one step at a time, and never mind what others think.

SELECTIONS THAT SATISFY

Part of the philosophy of listening to your body and tuning into taste and texture involves making gradual changes, one step at a time. If you are getting cravings for foods that are high in fat, it may be a sign that you are not eating frequently enough or that you are restricting your fat intake too much. You will gradually acquire a taste for new foods with lower fat content. Remember, the new way of eating is for life! You do not want to feel deprived while you are acquiring your new tastes.

You are listening to your body if:

- You are tuning into the texture, taste and satiety value of the meal.

- You are enjoying the energising feeling of balanced meals. Higher-fat meals make your mind and your body sluggish by slowing down circulation and reducing the oxygen-carrying capacity of the red blood cells. Meals that are too low in fat will leave you feeling hungry and thinking about food.

- You are accommodating your present taste preferences by making only slight changes in your eating pattern at a time.

- You are checking the regularity of meals and the type and quantity of food eaten if you are experiencing cravings.

- You are paying attention to the experience of eating and allowing yourself to taste, savour, and enjoy your meal.

If you answer no to some of the above questions, reassess whether you are eating too many low-fat foods and therefore need to readjust to a more normal and natural way of eating. A low-fat way of eating is not desirable for everyone all the time. If something does not feel right, make adjustments and go slower in the process of moving towards healthier eating. Recognise that any change is progress and that striving for a particular goal is falling back into the diet mentality. Use improved health as your guide. Tailor your tastes to appreciate the slight, subtle differences in the taste and texture of healthier foods. If they are not becoming choices you make because you prefer and enjoy them, then you are returning to the diet mentality.

If you need a snack, eat it or you will be too hungry by the next meal and will eat too quickly and not enjoy your food as much. Eat regularly, being guided by your physical hunger and appetite. Try introducing more carbohydrates, and do not restrict yourself to salads alone. They do not have much substance and may lead to binging later on. While a salad may fill you up more quickly because of the high water content of the lettuce, there is little substance and few nutrients in the meal. In fact, there is almost twice as much fat in a caesar salad as a roast beef sandwich. A meat sandwich, on the other hand, will provide you with more carbohydrate for energy, nutrients, and holding power, not to mention the feeling of satisfaction and taste. The aim is to focus more on the satisfaction, taste and 'holdover' power of foods and meals rather than on the content of fat and calories.

Compare fast food at home to a fast-food meal in a restaurant. A typical fast-food fried chicken dinner has over four times the amount of fat as a well-balanced twenty-minute home-made chicken dinner. Those of you familiar with fast-food fried chicken will remember the grease marks on plates and napkins, the greasy fingers and lips that require a soap and water wash after eating, the thirst produced by the extra salt needed to cut through the fat flavour, and the full and bloated feeling after eating. In contrast, the home-cooked chicken meal has a variety of colours, tastes, and textures and leaves a refreshing, satisfying feeling.

FAST FOOD AT HOME

Twenty-Minute Home-Cooked Chicken Dinner for Four
Baked Breaded Chicken
Rice
Peas with Green Onions
Sliced Tomato
Milk (semi-skimmed)

Compare this with:

Fast-Food Fried Chicken Dinner
1 piece side breast
Chips
Coleslaw
Milk (semi-skimmed)

TAKING THE FOCUS OFF FAT ADDS PIZZAZZ TO MEALS

'My partner is a great cook and it tastes so good. I agree with the saying "butter makes it better". Doesn't it?'

Maybe not. The true chef can use herbs tastefully without a lot of fat to bring out the flavours in a meal. Changing to a lower-fat way of eating can be a simple matter of adapting the foods you normally enjoy. Lower-fat eating can still mean eating very well, especially when foods are prepared at home. Food can be moist, tasty, and have flavour and texture without being heavy with grease.

In order to acquire a taste for foods and meals which are lower in fat you have to learn how to make gradual changes to your food preparation techniques so that you will enjoy the end product. The traditional way of frying with fat and no lid leads to moisture evaporation and food sticking to the bottom of the pan. Adding more fat results in a meal loaded with fat and grease, which is heavy on the stomach and difficult to digest. Instead of feeling energised, you feel drowsy.

Choosing meat with less marbling (the streaks of fat seen

throughout a cut of meat) and trimming all visible fat off meat before cooking can sometimes result in a drier, less tender product. Try using a non-stick frying pan with a lid to retain the moisture. Trim the fat from the meat, sear the meat in a non-stick frying pan with a light coating of oil, turn the meat over, brown, and add the lid while the meat cooks. When the oil has been heated, add onions, garlic, and fresh or dried herbs for more flavour prior to adding the meat. If the meat sticks to the pan, deglaze with wine, alcohol, milk, or vegetable or fruit juice, water and herbs, or broth or water with a stock cube to brown the meat nicely. The liquid will gradually evaporate and it can be thickened to make a gravy if desired. The alcoholic content does not remain.

You can brown meat in the oven instead of using a frying pan. Just coat the meat lightly with seasoned flour and place it on a rack set over a pan to catch the drippings. Bake at 350°F (180°C) for fifteen to twenty minutes. Chops can also be done in the oven on a rack in a covered dish. Add seasonings as desired.

Roasting can be done on a rack in a covered roaster. The rack prevents the fat drippings from coming into direct contact with the roast, so the roast will be less greasy. Use lower temperatures when cooking a roast, 325°F or 160°C (for tender cuts) and 275°F or 130°C (for medium tender cuts). This process retains the moisture, reduces shrinkage, and prevents the fat from going back into the roast. Gravy can be added for flavour, colour, and moisture. Remove the roast, then put ice cubes in the fat drippings to allow the drippings to cool quickly. The number of ice cubes added will depend on the volume of juices. Ensure that sufficient ice cubes are added so that all the fat rises to the top as it cools. Remove fat and thicken juices with flour or cornflour. Lump-free gravy thickeners are also available to make the job easier. Quark, yogurt, or oat bran can also be used as thickeners. Add extra seasonings such as garlic or onion powder or milder herbs and spices to add new flavours. Use sauces as accents to meat, not the main feature. Tune into texture and natural flavour. *Note* If time permits, placing the gravy in the freezer or fridge will allow the fat to float to the surface for easy removal.

Less tender cuts of meat are best cooked in liquid (braising, stewing, or pot roasting) to create succulent, tasty dishes.

Marinating meat helps to tenderise and add flavour. Marinating liquids include wine, vinegar, seasoned vinegars, soy sauce, citrus juices, beer, yogurt, and oil. The acidic ingredients soften the tough connective tissue and the oil lubricates. Often the oil can be eliminated. Don't use salt in a marinade because it draws out the moisture.

When microwaving beef, it is not recommended to bring the meat to room temperature before microwaving. It is best to slightly undercook beef. Remember, cooking continues during standing time. Large dense items need a standing time of ten to twenty minutes. Overcooking or cooking at too high a temperature causes the meat to be dry and tough.

Steaming, microwaving, or stir-frying vegetables retains their flavour, texture, and colour. If you sauté vegetables, cook them over a lower heat and add white wine or water to help soften them. The addition of fresh or dried herbs can heighten the flavour. Use herbs such as dill, rosemary, thyme, and garlic instead of salt for flavour. Thyme is a mild herb that works well with any dish and the bonus is that it is high in iron. *Note* To microwave your vegetables so they are crisp and not mushy, put a consistent quantity of vegetables cut uniformly on to a plate, cover with clingfilm and watch for it to fill with air. When this happens the vegetables are cooked but still crisp.

A small amount of a simple white sauce will enhance the natural flavour of vegetables.

White sauce Place one teaspoon (five ml) of oil in a non-stick frying pan. Add fresh or dried herbs to hot oil to extract the flavour of the herbs. Add chopped onions, if desired. Add skimmed or semi-skimmed milk or yogurt and heat. Thicken with flour or cornflour, or for convenience add white instant gravy thickener. If you prefer a cheese sauce, add a hint of your favourite cheese to accent the flavour of the vegetables (too much cheese will mask the taste of the vegetables).

When using oil to sauté foods, use a heavy, non-stick pan so that a light coating of oil will prevent the food burning. Make sure the oil is hot before adding the ingredients in order to reduce the amount of oil that soaks into the food.

Chips   Crisp, tasty chips can be made without them tasting and feeling greasy. Cut potatoes into wedges, toss in a little oil to coat the potatoes lightly, and add seasoning if desired. Cook in a hot oven (425° to 450°F; 210° to 230°C) on a non-stick baking tray brushed with a very thin coating of oil to prevent the potatoes from sticking as the starch is released. Cook for fifteen to twenty-five minutes, turn and cook for another fifteen to twenty-five minutes, or until brown. *Note* Potatoes do not need to be peeled. Peel adds colour and fibre to the potatoes. Most of the vitamins are right under the peel and it is a shame to throw them away. Add paprika or your favourite seasoning. These potatoes are a real treat for the whole family.

Savoury rice   The cooking instructions on the rice packet may call for butter or margarine. Since easy-cook rice is so overly processed it needs extra fat or spices to give it flavour. Use converted rice instead. It takes only twenty minutes to cook, has more nutrients than even long grain rice, and you end up with rice that does not stick together. Add a stock cube or juice to the water to add flavour to the rice. Chopped vegetables such as celery, mushrooms, onions, and herbs and spices make a very nice rice pilaf. Brown rice is now available in the converted form (the rice is parboiled and some of the nutrients are pushed back in). Note that packaged savoury rice is costly and is often disappointing and artificial tasting, so go with the real thing!

Flavour enhancers   Herbs and spices are natural flavour enhancers. Substitutes for high-fat products are effective only if you enjoy the replacement. For example, if you enjoy butter on your baked potato and you replace it with a lower-fat product such as light sour cream or yogurt, which you don't really like, then eventually you will crave the butter. The true butter connoisseur might try gradually using less butter as an accent to the meal. A small amount of the real thing may be more satisfying than a large amount of something artificial. On the other hand, if you enjoy the replacement, then the substitute will work. Low-fat substitutes, such as diet margarines or diet butters, are high in water content. For this reason, they cannot be used for frying. If you try to fry with them, you will notice that the pan soon becomes dry because the water from the product evaporates as soon as it is exposed to heat. The high water content of these products can make hot toast soggy. Experiment and do what works best for you.

If you are drinking full cream milk, try diluting it with semi-skimmed for a week or two until you get accustomed to this taste. Then try semi-skimmed milk for a week or two. Work your way down to mixing semi-skimmed and skimmed, and then finally switch to skimmed. Skimmed milk has a fuller body than it did years ago. As you become aware you will gradually acquire a taste for foods with a more refreshing, lighter texture. This is much easier and more enjoyable than the diet approach of going from whole milk to skimmed milk in one fell swoop.

Cheese has a high hidden fat content. If you like cheddar cheese and go straight to cottage cheese, you may find it difficult to adjust to this sudden drop in fat content. If you don't like cottage cheese because of its taste and lumpy texture, then you will eat it temporarily because you think you should and then go back to what you were doing before. If you prefer the taste and texture of cheddar cheese, try mixing it with low-fat mozzarella to gradually reduce the greasy texture but still savour the cheddar taste. Eventually you may prefer the lighter taste of low-fat mozzarella.

Why There Aren't Numbers (Calories or Fat Counts) in This Book

Focusing on numbers can take the enjoyment out of life and it doesn't help us to become healthier, happier people. We exercise to lose weight or burn calories rather than to enjoy the outdoors or feel the improved energy and self-image that activity brings. We feel good about ourselves on the days when we weigh the 'right' amount and feel depressed and forlorn when we are above that weight. Often we choose foods because they are lower in fat or have fewer calories rather than because we enjoy them. But when we get tired of counting we crave the familiar flavours, tastes, and activities we enjoyed before, and we return to our old eating habits and patterns. None of these numbers help us to become healthy and numbers don't help us to learn to enjoy the flavours and textures of foods which are lower in fat, sugar, and salt and higher in fibre. Numbers just provide a rule book of what is 'good' and 'bad' to eat.[8]

So let's look at food in another way. What are the flavours and textures of the foods we enjoy? What is it about food that we enjoy? Can we slowly change our preference for familiar flavours and textures to reflect healthier eating patterns without becoming obsessed with numbers? We know we can! The chart on this page illustrates how the tastes and textures of familiar foods prepared and served in the usual ways can slowly be replaced by an appreciation of foods and meals with more refreshing and energising qualities. It isn't important to know the exact calorie or fat content of food. What is important is that you enjoy what you eat.[9]

THE PROCESS OF TAILORING YOUR TASTES

Traditional	New Experience
Appearance	
Grease may be seen or is floating on top of sauces, salads or soups. Washed out colours of vegetables. Thick beverages. Grease leaves a mark on napkins.	Refreshing, clean looking. Sauces, dressings, and garnishes provide a colourful accent without overwhelming the food. Exciting colours and textures.
Taste	
Subtle flavours not noticeable. Flavours masked by fat taste. Sauce, dressing or garnish overwhelms the food. Needs more salt or sugar to bring out flavours masked by fat.	Natural flavour can be tasted. Less salt and seasoning needed. The more you taste it, the better it gets; taste is subtle and builds gradually. Sauces, dressings and garnishes enhance flavour without overwhelming it.
Texture	
Mushy, gooey, soft, dense, greasy.	Crunchy, crisp, chewy, cleaner.
Oral response	
Coats mouth, greasy; beverages leave mouth dry, coated with fullness of beverage.	Experience the variety of texture and consistencies. Beverages feel refreshing and go down easily.
Body response	
Heavy feeling as it goes down. Feel tired and bloated when finished. Beverages leave you still feeling thirsty.	Refreshing, satisfying feeling as it goes down. Not overfilling. Leaves you energised. Beverages quench your thirst.

Tailoring your tastes to enjoy new flavours and textures is a slow, pleasurable process. Over time, your new choices will become preferences. You will choose cooking techniques and foods that are lower in fat, sugar and salt, and higher in fibre because you prefer them, not because you think you should eat them. When you prefer something, you repeat it. Repeating healthier lifestyle practices leads to healthier living. You can find more information regarding these areas in *Tailoring Your Tastes*.[10]

MODIFYING RECIPES TO SUIT YOUR NEW TASTES

Getting in tune with the YCCD philosophy does not mean turning to special low-fat versions of recipes and spending a lot of time preparing new foods. It means modifying your present recipes and learning what you can do to enjoy new flavours and textures which are not masked by fat. Use your own recipes, and let your creativity and new-found knowledge allow you to make slight changes so that you produce food which is moist, tasty and lower in fat and sugar content.

Muffins
The fat provides moisture and flavour while the sugar acts as a tenderiser and sweetener. The recipe needs sugar for the egg to coagulate at a higher temperature, allowing the muffins to rise. Cutting out the sugar completely will result in small muffins.

Initially decrease the sugar and fat in the recipe by a quarter. Next time you make muffins, you may be able to decrease the sugar and fat a little more. Enhance the new flavours by using sweeter spices such as cinnamon, mace, lemon extract, vanilla extract, lemon or orange peel, or your favourite spice. If the recipe already contains one of these, try doubling the amount.

Retain the moisture by adding milk, yogurt, or light sour cream. Apple sauce, pineapple, fruit juice, blueberries, shredded carrots, or chopped raisins can add back moisture and some sweetness. Raisins are a concentrated source of sugar so a small amount goes a long way.

To make the muffins rise, add baking powder and baking soda to the sifted flour (half a teaspoon or two ml of baking soda and two teaspoons or ten ml of baking powder). Ensure that you sift the baking powder and baking soda with the flour, otherwise lumps of these ingredients may appear in your muffins. If you can taste the soda and do not like it, then add a little more sugar the next time and cut back slightly on the baking soda in the recipe.

Biscuits

The fat allows the creaming effect of the ingredients and provides flavour. The sugar provides sweetness and also helps the creaming effect.

Sugar, flour, and fat are the main ingredients. Cutting back on sugar and fat too much does not allow the creaming effect to occur. Sugar also adds to the sweetness of the biscuits so you may be able to cut back by about half and replace with some sweeter spices such as nutmeg and cinnamon. Fat content can only be cut back slightly (by about a quarter). Cutting the fat content too much will change the nature of the recipe. A crispy oatmeal biscuit may become a chewy oatmeal bar that, with time, will go hard. To keep biscuits moist, add milk to replace the moisture taken out by cutting back the fat content. Apple sauce or blueberries can also add back moisture to biscuits or brownies. Try storing biscuits in an airtight tin with a slice of apple. This will help to retain some moisture.

The idea is to modify your present recipes so that they still taste good and you will enjoy them. The purpose is to learn to taste and savour more wholesome foods. Learn to tune into the texture and wholesome flavour and ensure that the end product is enjoyable.

Cakes or Quick Breads

Try replacing the butter in your recipe with sour cream. If this works, the next step is to replace the sour cream with plain low-fat yogurt.

Use the concept of replacing oil with fruit juice to give moisture and flavour to all your cooking. Chicken fingers made this way are moist and tasty. Use a deboned chicken breast, dunk slices in concentrated orange juice and then bread crumbs or crushed cornflakes. Bake in the oven. Makes a tasty meal or an innovative snack! Let your creativity take hold and create your own recipes.

ACTION POINTS

● Notice and appreciate tastes and textures of particular foods.

● What gradual changes to your eating patterns can you make so that your food still leaves you satisfied and the changes will last? For example, don't cut out butter if you love it. Try to gradually reduce the amount.

● Begin moderating your favourite recipes by using herbs, spices and fruit juices to flavour your food, and gradually replace fatty ingredients.

● Think and write down ways to develop a taste for foods which are lower in fat, such as:

using fat as an accent instead of masking the true flavour and texture of food;

tailoring your tastes to slide smoothly into healthier eating instead of jumping straight in (moving straight into low-fat eating is diet thinking); and

tasting the difference little changes make as you decrease the fat content of your meals one step at a time (by eating less processed foods, buying leaner cuts of meat, experimenting with cooking methods that require less fat yet retain moisture and flavour).

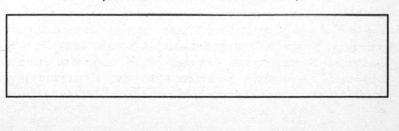

6

When to Eat, How Much to Eat

Tune into your natural hunger signals. Eat whatever you want whenever you want, as long as you are physically hungry.

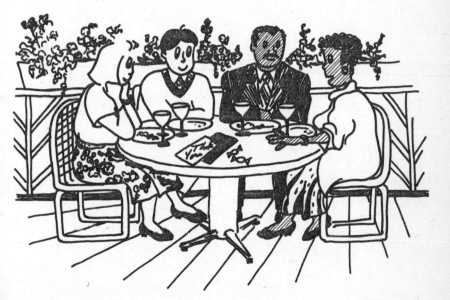

THE FREEDOM OF NO SET DIET

The positive result of a lack of structure is flexibility. You can replace your old way of eating with an improved and healthier way of eating. If you have been accustomed to following a diet, you may think that this method cannot work since there is no rigid pattern to follow. However, focus and flexibility can replace structure.

The focus is getting you to deal with the cause of your poor eating habits. Why did you get to this stage in the first place? The focus is to show you how to eat in a way that gives you more energy and keeps you satisfied.

Follow our guidelines and balance your carbohydrates and protein sources, gradually cut back the fat content in your food choices and cooking methods, and note when you are actually physically hungry. If you eat all the time, you won't give your body a chance to experience hunger. If you are used to dieting and starving, you may be out of tune with what real hunger is, especially if you have been ignoring it for a number of years. If you have recently stopped smoking, you too will be out of touch with your internal hunger signals. If you wait until you are too hungry, there is a danger of being famished, 'gobbling' your food, and overeating. In these situations it's unlikely that you are tasting your food.

This programme gives you permission to eat. The danger is that you may swing the other way and eat everything in sight. Can this happen? Long-term denial and deprivation of food can lead to a rebellion against dieting, whether you or someone else gives you the permission to eat. Permission to eat can be frightening because of the lack of rigid control. Now you are taking charge. Rather than someone else learning to ride the bike for you, you are actually learning to ride it yourself. You are learning a new skill.

When you feel you can't or shouldn't have something, you

often desire it more. On the other hand, if you know you can have it, you might not want it as much. Realise that you are striving to bring the pendulum back to the middle so that you learn to eat like a non-dieter, that is, someone who eats when he or she is physically hungry. Check how you feel three to four hours after eating to help you tune into your natural hunger.

DO DIETERS THINK DIFFERENTLY?

Do you think like a non-dieter? Two psychologists, Polivy and Herman, from Toronto,[1] gave forty dieters and forty non-dieters two milkshakes each to drink followed by an offer of ice cream as part of a controlled study.

The dieters finished their milkshakes and ate the ice cream too. The non-dieters ate very little ice cream once they finished the milkshakes. Why is there a difference between the actions of the dieters and the non-dieters? The dieters' thinking is all-or-nothing thinking. 'I blew my diet anyway, so I'll go for it and eat it all. Since I'll go back to dieting and depriving myself tomorrow, I'd better get my fill.' Dieters either diet faithfully or not at all. Once they have been deprived for so long, they may not be able to control themselves. The pendulum has swung the other way.

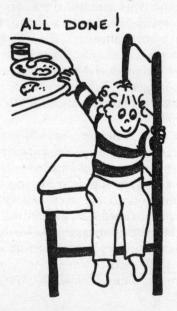

Dieters are often perfectionists and their 'absolutely perfect' mentality transfers to other aspects of their life as well. 'I'll clean the house completely or not at all. I'm that type of person.' It is this all-or-nothing thinking that can lead to frustration when something doesn't proceed perfectly. This type of rigid thinking does not allow a person to be human.

There is flexibility in the non-dieter's thinking and this is how it differs from the dieter's thinking. The non-dieters, once the milkshakes were finished, chose to eat very little ice cream because they were in tune with their bodies' feelings of hunger and fullness. They were satisfied with the milkshakes and were no longer hungry. The added fact that they knew they could have more ice cream when they wanted it decreased the need to have it immediately. The non-dieters were tuning into their internal cues of hunger. The dieters responded to the external cue of sight. 'I see it – I want it!' Continue to observe non-dieters and children. They are in tune with their natural hunger signals and those that signal appetite and fullness (physical satisfaction). Note what they do in order to eat when they are hungry and stop when they are full, and try to model their actions.

The second part of the Polivy and Herman study dealt with both groups being given no milkshakes, after which both groups were offered ice cream. This time the dieters ate no ice cream. The 'all-or-nothing' response was 'I'm still on my diet, so since I did not start to eat anything illegal, I'll be able to forgo the ice cream. I have the willpower to say no.' The non-dieters who did not have milkshakes but were offered ice cream ate a lot of ice cream. They were tuning into their internal hunger signals. The non-dieters were physically hungry and therefore ate the offered ice cream.

How do you shift your thinking to be a non-dieter? The first step is to acknowledge what you are doing and accept it, just as you accepted yourself as you are unconditionally. Without self-acceptance, too much energy is diverted towards feeling sorry for yourself and feeling negative.

An illustration of this is a neglected plant that grows tall, thin, and straggly as the energy is diverted upwards. With a little caring, by pruning it, the energy is no longer wasted but rather the nutrients and energy are used where they are most needed, for growth. By accepting yourself, you use your energy to take care of yourself rather than divert your energy by criticising yourself.

We want you to grow from within and burst forth with new shoots, as the plant does. So don't waste your energy being negative. Go with the flow and learn from your mistakes. Care about yourself enough to listen to your body and find out what is really causing you to eat. Ask yourself what is happening that you need to distract yourself by eating or worrying about your eating? Take a moment to reflect on the reasons why you are eating.

DIET THINKING	NON-DIET THINKING
'all-or-nothing'	listens to the body's needs
I will have it all or nothing at all	is flexible
perfectionist attitude	human – goes with the flow
responds to external cues of sight, smell, and power of suggestion	responds to internal cues – eats when hungry
out of touch with physical hunger – may eat in response to psychological hunger, i.e. when under stress	in tune with body's internal cues of physical hunger; listens to body, does not turn to food when dealing with problems such as stress
diet is in control	person is in control and decides when and what to eat
asks self, 'Should I have it, do I need it?'	asks self, 'Do I want it?'

Reasons for eating:

- boredom;
- loneliness;
- frustration;
- stress;
- anger;

- rushed;

- comfort food;

- tension;

- social occasion;

- everyone else is eating;

- happy;

- sad;

- 'see-food' diet ('I see it, I want it');

- tired;

- insomnia;

- PMS.

When you eat for these reasons, are you really tasting your food or are you eating to drown sorrows? Does food give you a temporary lift? Does it deal with the problem? It's time to replace this dependency on food. Have confidence in yourself, trust yourself, believe in yourself. Only you can uncover the reasons for your eating and learn new techniques to deal with them more positively. Remember that if you feel you were not successful in the past, it is not you that failed but the diets that failed you. **Diets don't work.** You can succeed by getting rid of the diet and the diet mentality. As you begin to discover yourself, you will be drawing on your inner self, that is, you will be internally motivated. Remember, action creates motivation. Once you have discovered why you are eating, take action.

Now that you have discovered why you are eating, what do you do about it? Meet the causes of your eating head on. Eating only provides temporary relief from thinking about your other problems. These problems will recur if you don't deal with them, and so will the eating. Catch yourself as you are reaching for the food and ask yourself, 'Do I really want it or do I think I want it simply because it's there and everyone else is eating?' If you just follow the crowd then the calories are wasted and will end up on your waist. Part of lifestyle change is acquiring a taste for less fattening foods and learning to eat until you are satisfied, not stuffed. Eat only those things that you really want and only if you are hungry.

When you eat because of a happy event to celebrate something that you accomplished, the food becomes a reward. It is a social custom to eat at such times and this is why you feel that you need something as an external reward to complete the happiness. Try not eating and allow yourself to experience the pleasant feeling of accomplishment for itself.

Eating because you are sad, depressed, or angry may provide a temporary comfort that you are searching for. But the problem that brought on these feelings remains and must be dealt with. Do you feel that you must always be 'up' and happy? What's wrong with allowing yourself to experience sad or frustrating emotions and working them through? It is part of normal life to go through these 'ups and downs'. Try to deal with the issues at hand. This will help to level off the roller coaster ride of emotions.

Loneliness, boredom, and television seem to trigger the food munchies. Social occasions where there is drinking also empties many peanut bowls. Suddenly you are out of control, the peanut bowl is empty, and you don't even remember eating them. Loneliness is often tied to not fully appreciating our own company. Nancy always goes into the 'tea and toast' syndrome when her husband is away. After all, she has no one to cook for or to try to please. She reaches for the sweets to keep her company and to comfort her.

Wait a minute! You are worth the little extra effort to prepare a sit-down meal for yourself, and maybe even a candle to go with it. This is your free time; you can do whatever you want. It's your own free time; you can do whatever you want. It's your own time to reassess your goals and redirect your life, time to think things through or maybe just relax, clear your mind and enjoy some peaceful moments. Don't waste the moment by feeling sorry for yourself. You are special too!

You come home from work, tired. You eat, clean up, and then plonk yourself in front of the television. There is nothing else to do so you might as well eat. Stimulation is in order. People tend to get into an everyday humdrum routine, taking the safe and easy route in life. Well, this route is also the boring route. Try to incorporate a little risk, a little excitement, a little adventure into your life. One of my favourite years of married life was the year we didn't have a television. We made our own fun and enjoyed simple things. Sure we need goals and direction to get somewhere in life, but we also need to make room for spontaneity and fun – even a little adventure now and then! When we grow up, we become more serious about life. Observe children once in a while and then attempt to bring out the child in you.

Overeating at social occasions once in a while isn't an issue. It's part of being normal. The type of thinking to watch out for is dieting during the week, only to allow yourself to binge on the weekend. This is the diet mentality. Try eating the foods you desire more regularly, then when someone offers your favourite onion rings, you can eat a few and not crave them so much that you stuff yourself. Taste and savour and enjoy without guilt and you will be satisfied with less. You may slip back into the diet thinking from time to time. After all, it was part of you for many years. But if you are aware of this, you can overcome it.

If you can't sleep at night unless you get up for biscuits and milk perhaps you should go to bed hungry. One of my clients, Betty, frequently had trouble sleeping. At two o'clock in the morning she got up for her snack and then went to sleep. Avoiding a snack before bedtime did not help her reduce her overall calorie intake. It prevented her from sleeping and she had to have a snack at an inconvenient time of the morning. If it has been over three to four hours since you ate supper, consider a little snack before going to bed. A small snack will not ruin your hunger for breakfast the next morning.

Experiment and Find Out What Works Best for You. Listen to Your Body!
Karen was tired early in the evening but believed that she could stay up with the rest of the family. She ate to keep herself awake. Since she physically had no energy, she attempted to retrieve energy from food. Perhaps Karen's best action would be to go to bed early once in a while and realise that it is normal to be tired on some days. However, if the tired feeling persists, she should make an attempt to incorporate more activity and regular meals into her eating pattern to give her energy level a boost!

Enough sleep is essential. It's a basic physiological need. Being sleep-deprived is not an indication of strong character or willpower. It is harmful to your health. Yet in this fast-paced, competitive society, sleep is often undermined and sacrificed. It's considered a waste of time in an age when people are valued for what they do, not who they are. The danger is that we may become workaholics, attaching our self-worth to tremendous achievements. Our goals may be impossible as we're driven to prove ourselves, to be dynamic with boundless energy. This affects our mental health, sleep, and eating patterns.

Learn to take everything a step at a time. Keep your goals within comfortable reach and build in balance along the way. Be satisfied to be the best you can be and don't push yourself beyond your capacity.

If your schedule is so busy that you can't take time for a meal, bring along handy snacks such as cheese, crackers, bread, rolls, fruit, or yogurt. Healthy snacks are not only a wise alternative to a skipped meal, but they can help you make the transition to taking the time to eat. Building in some relaxing 'time out' from your rushed schedule gives you a chance to nourish your body and refuel your energy reserves. Your productivity will increase because you will be more alert. You will have a clear mind to keep you working those extra hours. Try it and feel the difference! Pausing to eat can help you to deal with stressful situations better than when your blood sugar level is low.

Sufficient restful sleep, proper nutrition, physical activity, relaxation, building in time for yourself, and knowing when to pull back helps you to deal with stress more easily. Ignoring your body's signals and not taking care of it may result in burn out and time off work. Think about it and re-adjust your lifestyle accordingly.

If you eat when you are under stress this kind of eating is strictly automatic. You are trying to solve your problem while eating and you are definitely not focusing on the food. Once again, wasted calories are ingested. Dealing with the issue is the way forward for you.

Pre-menstrual syndrome known as PMS is a normal biological occurrence that bothers many women prior to the onset of their menstrual period. Realise that you may be hungrier more frequently due to the rise in progesterone which causes the level of your blood sugar to drop. Because of this, hunger strikes more often. The answer is to eat more frequently, and understand that giving in to those cravings for caffeine in the form of chocolate or coffee may aggravate your blood sugar swings.

Don't deny yourself the foods you like. You can leave room for these foods, but you will have them on a fuller stomach rather than an empty one. If you have these cravings, you may simply be hungry. Don't ignore your natural hunger signals that occur more frequently during this time of the month. Stay tuned to your body's changing needs and observe them in order to find out what your body needs. The 'I see it, I want it' mentality will occur less frequently as you switch into non-diet thinking and normalise your eating and lifestyle habits.

Try to get rid of the diet mentality and learn to think like a non-dieter. If you like butter don't deny yourself. When Donna replaced butter with margarine, she initially used less, because she didn't like the taste. Eventually, she felt deprived. Once she resumed eating butter she binged on it. Donna's diet thinking, which demanded substitution of foods with less enticing items, was wrong for her. Dieters feel that if they don't like the substituted food, they won't eat as much. That may be true temporarily, but eventually the dieter feels deprived and binges on the forbidden food.

Fat adds flavour but tends to take away the texture by making the food soggy. You can experience both. Use a little less butter and eventually you will enjoy the real taste of bread without the grease. Experimenting with different types of whole grain breads will allow you to discover a new dimension in eating. Or add a protein source to give you some moisture and more nutrient content with fewer 'fat' calories.

Take the case of nine-year-old Paul who butters his toast only in the centre because that's the way he likes it. Along comes Mum who says, 'No, no, Paul, that's not the way you butter toast. Spread the butter out to the sides, otherwise it will be too hard.' Like Paul, most children naturally have a taste for less fattening foods until we as parents impose our own preferences on them – just as our parents did to us.

Try to acquire a taste for baked potato with butter rather

than butter with the baked potato. You can use substitutes (margarine), but margarine contains the same number of fat calories. Sour cream is a lower fat choice. But if you really miss the butter, then use it and gradually decrease the quantity. Within a few months, you will enjoy your potato with less total fat content and not feel deprived. Gradually you will acquire a taste for less fattening foods. Low-fat gravy is also an excellent choice. It is full of flavour. Experience it and you may be converted!

The diet mentality of all-or-nothing thinking instead of gradual change hampers the progress you are making. Debbie had a sandwich for lunch without chips and then had a chocolate bar. She thought that she had failed because she gave in to her craving. But it was the time of the month when her hormonal change caused her to crave chocolate. On pursuing this instance, we discovered that normally Debbie would have eaten a sandwich and chips followed by two chocolate bars. She realised that she was making progress! Note the positive changes you are making. When you occasionally fall into the all-or-nothing thinking, don't be too hard on yourself.

Get your mind into gear and shift into thinking like a non-dieter. What about those chocolate almonds or sweets that you cannot refuse at a party? Other people take one or two and are satisfied. Why can't you? Have you been denying yourself these foods, regarding them as special treats only to be eaten at certain special occasions? Remember that denial leads to the eventual binge. Do you really taste these chocolates or is it automatic eating? You may be eating them for one of the following reasons:

- because they are there, an external cue;

- because you think you may not have them again for a while; or

- because it's a special occasion so it's all right to eat on a special occasion.

Dieters have difficulty distinguishing between 'should', 'need', and 'want'. Dieters may feel that they always want a dessert after a meal because it is part of the meal. Habit may be confused with the real desire to have it. However, realising that you can have it later on and accepting this fact will help to clarify the difference between 'want' and 'need'. Just because it is there and you see it is no reason to eat it. Eat it only if you are physically hungry for the food.

Should I have the biscuit? Do I need it? These questions reflect the diet thinking. Replacing this question with 'Do I want the biscuit?' gets you on the road to non-diet thinking.

Phyllis, when on a diet, used to eat the raw cake mixture when she was making cakes because the finished product was on her 'illegal' list of foods. With her new way of thinking, she allows herself to have the cakes but often chooses not to, simply because she doesn't want them at the time. After all, she can have them later on if she wants. What a relief to no longer have that mental struggle with food!

If, after using these techniques for a while, you still feel the urge to eat the entire tin of cakes, you may still be partly in the diet thinking. You may feel you want them but are still getting mixed signals. When confronting the urge to eat a particular food, practise your new skills in non-stressful situations so that you allow this powerful skill to work for you when you need it. Being preoccupied with confrontation does not allow it to happen naturally. To help it happen naturally, ask yourself 'Do I really want it or do I think I want it because it's there and I like it (partly out of habit)? I know I can have it later on if I want it. And if it is no longer there, I can buy or make some more.'

WHAT DOES IT MEAN TO FEEL HUNGRY?

What does it mean to feel hungry? What does it mean to eat till you're satisfied and not overly full? Once again, observe non-dieters and notice what they do to tune into their natural hunger signals. To begin to eat normally and think as non-dieters do, who eat when they are hungry and stop when they are full:

- Ask yourself, 'Am I eating because I really want it or because I feel it will no longer be there tomorrow?' Eating 'normally' for most dieters suggests being 'off the diet'. They think they have to 'stuff it in' before going on a diet again. Tell yourself, 'I don't have to overeat. It will be there later on.'

- Ask yourself, 'Am I eating because it is there and I see it (automatic eating) or do I really want it?' If you are not tasting and savouring your food and consciously eating it, then it is 'waisted' calories. Tell yourself, 'I want it only if I am physically hungry. If I eat for other reasons, I will not focus on my food while eating, tasting, and savouring my food without guilt. In this way, I will eat less food and 'waist' fewer calories.'

- Ask yourself, 'If I eat a piece of cake because I want it, and I can't stop at one piece, what is happening when I lose control?' Perhaps you think you want the piece of cake simply because you haven't eaten for a while and your blood sugar level is low (this means you are hungry). Tell yourself, 'This is a normal reaction. I will eat when I am pleasantly hungry. Waiting until I am too hungry causes me to desire the quick sugar and to overeat on these foods.'

Eating regularly keeps you from binging because of insatiable hunger. Often people binge for a number of reasons, either because they have been deprived or because they allow themselves to get too hungry.

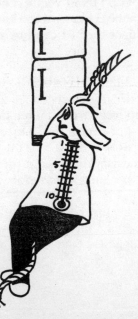

Let's look at a scale of hunger that will help you to determine what it really means to feel physically hungry. We suggest that you do not let yourself get past number 3 on the scale (p164). At that point you no longer care what you are eating as long as you are fed. Aim to eat to keep your blood sugar away from the 'hills' and 'valleys' that can occur with improperly balanced eating habits. YCCD shows you how to eat so that you can get more sustained energy from foods. It advocates the balance of carbohydrate and protein that allows the sugar to be released into your bloodstream at a more gradual rate. In this way, physical hunger will not overtake you so quickly. When you eat balanced meals (a balance between carbohydrate and protein), physical hunger will not set in for three to six hours after a meal.

If your hunger level is under 5, you are consuming food as a fuel source and feeding your physical hunger. If you are above 5 you are dealing with the social pressure to eat. This psychological eating feeds the head rather than the body and you are no longer in control.

One of my clients was a constant nibbler. She never gave herself a chance to get hungry. By allowing more time between eating, she discovered what it feels like to be hungry. On the other hand, if you diet below your weight set point (the point your body deems normal for you), you may always be hungry. It's your body's way of protecting you from going below your natural weight. The starvation way of losing weight seems to trigger the body to binge as a protective measure to bring the body weight back to normal or the set point. This method of starving and binging does not allow you to tune into your internal hunger signals. *Note* Before shopping for food, eat a snack if your meal will be delayed. Shopping when hungry can easily run up your bill on high-sugar, high-fat foods. These are particularly tempting when your blood sugar is low.

HUNGER LEVEL SCALE

1 1 You may have a headache. You can't think straight and feel dizzy. You may have trouble with coordination. You are totally out of energy and need to lie down. This may happen on the first day of a starvation diet.

2 2 You can't seem to tolerate anything. You have a short fuse. You're irritable and cranky and very hungry but have little energy. Your stomach may be rumbling giving you the signal to eat. You may even feel nauseous. You are at the stage of being famished.

3 3 The urge to eat is strong. You are feeling an emptiness in your stomach. Your concentration begins to wane.

4 You start to think about food. Your body is giving you the signal that you might want to eat. You are a little hungry.

4 4.9 Your hunger is almost gone. You're just a couple of mouthfuls away from feeling satisfied, without loosening the belt.

5 5 The non-dieter stops eating here. Your body has enough fuel to keep it going and is physically and psychologically satisfied. You are not hungry anymore.

5.1 You are eating more than your body needs for fuel. You are beginning to feed your psychological hunger. Did you not taste and savour your meal and focus on the meal while you were eating?

6 6 You're past the point of satisfaction, yet you could still eat more. Your body says 'no' and your mind says 'yes' to a few more bites so you eat past the point of physical hunger.

7 7 Here comes the loosening of the belt. You're beginning to feel uncomfortable. You feel bloated.

8 8 You are past the point of feeling full. You are actually starting to hurt. Maybe you shouldn't have had more but it tasted so good. Or did you get caught up in the eating-is-the-thing-to-do syndrome because all activity was centred around food?

9 9 The after-effects really hurt. You didn't eat all day to leave room for this meal and you packed it in. You feel heavy, tired, bloated. You no longer feel like socialising; you'd rather go home to bed. Did you miss out on the true meaning of the occasion because you were too centred on food?

10 10 This is holiday time. It starts in December and goes on until Christmas and New Year. It's socially acceptable to stuff yourself on holiday occasions. But now you are paying the price for it. You ate so much that you roll over to the sofa after dinner and tell yourself that you won't eat for another week. You really overdid it this time!

ACTION POINTS

- Check how you feel three to four hours after eating.

- Give yourself permission to eat. Remember, deprivation leads to binging, a normal response to the deprivation process.

- Eat whatever you want, whenever you want – when you are physically hungry.

- Photocopy the hunger scale: post in the kitchen, have a copy with you if it will help you tune in and listen to your body. This is your guide to what hunger is.

- Observe the way children and non-dieters eat. Model their actions. Dieters respond to external cues. Non-dieters listen to their internal cues of hunger.

- Tune into your needs for certain foods. Ask yourself, 'Do I want it?', not 'Should I have it?' or 'Do I need it?'

- Practise listening to your body to differentiate between your physical and psychological hunger.

- Is there anything more you need to do to ensure you are getting enough sleep, nutrition, physical activity, and relaxation? Make a note of your ideas.

- If PMS is an issue for you read p158 again and put into practice.

7

Automatic Eating: How to Take Charge

Eat until you are physically satisfied, not overly full

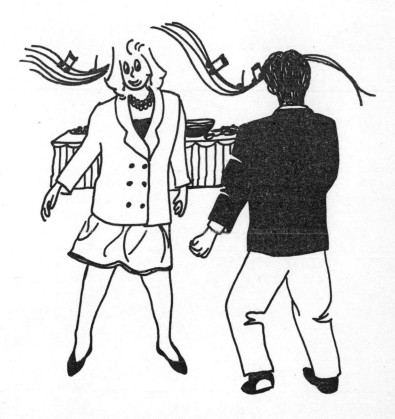

Automatic eating refers to eating that occurs unconsciously. Suddenly, the packet of biscuits has gone and you didn't even realise it. Studies have shown that urges to overeat are like waves, they gradually build, peak, and then decline. When you have an urge to eat, note whether it is actually physical hunger because you have not eaten for a while or perhaps it is for one of the other reasons discussed in the previous chapter.

People often feel the social pressure to eat when they go to visit someone. They eat to be sociable or polite, rather than to satisfy their hunger. People with low self-esteem need to find acceptance by pleasing others. Ask yourself if you are overeating simply because everyone else is eating, or if you really want to eat because you are hungry.

Studies have shown that the most satisfaction from eating comes from the first and last few bites and that the middle bites are automatic. This means that you eat the middle bites because they are there, not because you are actually tasting and savouring the food. These calories pile on to your waist and the food is not really being tasted. Does this just translate into cutting back and taking a smaller portion?

Bonnie walked into an ice cream parlour with a couple of friends who were on diets. She wanted a sundae so she ordered one. Her friends, on the other hand, may have yearned for one but, since they were on diets, they chose not to have one. Bonnie enjoyed the treat without guilt. She tasted and savoured it and then a third of the way through she was satisfied and she left it unfinished. She knew she could have another sundae any time she wished so she had no need to binge.

Why did she leave part of it? Not because she felt pressured. Not because she had to eat in moderation and cut quantities. If you remember the Polivy and Herman examples from Chapter 6, dieters, once they start eating something, cannot stop until it is finished. Dieters say, 'I blew my diet anyway so I might as well eat the whole thing and diet tomorrow.' Or dieters may eat the treat with guilt or in secrecy or too fast, and not feel totally satisfied, ending up binging on another sundae. Or they may eat several because of the feeling of being deprived. My client was exhibiting the non-diet mentality. She no longer felt satisfaction from the sundae so she left it. It is true that the most satisfaction comes from the first few bites because you look forward to the taste, and the last few bites because you won't have it again for a while. The middle bites give you no great satisfaction. They are eaten by dieters because of the external cue of seeing the food. Non-dieters are selective and eat only what they really want.

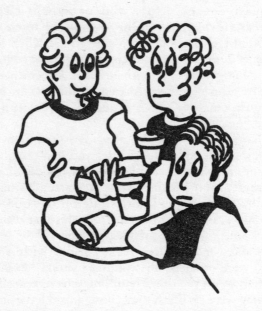

What did the dieters who just ordered coffee or diet drinks do when they got home? They binged on everything in sight. They felt deprived and they wanted the sundae but it was an illegal food for the diet. When they got home they tried to find something that would satisfy their craving for a sweet. Usually these people eat more calories in the replacement food than if they had eaten the sundae. For them, **calories don't count if no one else sees you eat it.** This is diet thinking that contributes to you eating more, not less. Dieters end up denying themselves on the one hand and hanging on the fridge door later on.

Constant calorie restriction followed by binging on foods plays havoc with your metabolic rate. Every time you starve and binge, your metabolic rate drops, which means that fewer calories will be burned at rest. It is essential to cut back gradually rather than suddenly on your total fat intake. Otherwise, you will be treating this programme as a diet where changes are drastic and temporary. If you do this, the effect will be to lower your metabolic rate as it responds to the sudden shock to your system caused by being deprived of the usual number of calories.

You want permanent change, and your tastes can change only if you introduce new things gradually. This allows you to make healthy choices because of your new preferences, not because it is on your diet sheet. What a difference in thinking! Even if you have never dieted before, you may be partially in the diet mentality because of being influenced by society's preoccupation with food and weight. 'I'll have it but I really shouldn't. I'll diet tomorrow.' Slimmer people may not necessarily be healthy. Many starve and binge to maintain the desired figure or they are constantly on and off diets.

Change in thinking is crucial to long-term success. Eating in a healthy manner because you 'have to' or are on a diet offers only a temporary solution because you are not in control. When you are not in control the changes won't be permanent. Making gradual changes allows you to acquire a taste for less fattening foods. In this way your preferences change, causing your choices to change. Food changes are based on cultivated preferences rather than rigid self-control.

Giving yourself permission to eat, using guidelines to help you retrieve more energy from foods will allow sweets to lose their appeal. When you realise that you don't have to give up sweets but can have them when you want, then eating only a bite or two to get the satisfaction from the food becomes easier. You need to trust yourself to take charge, to make choices, to enjoy your life. If you believe you are in charge you will be.

Your non-diet thinking will allow you to have a chocolate bar if you really want it. By tasting and savouring the bar and eating it without guilt, you will probably be satisfied with less. However, because of the high caffeine and sugar content of a chocolate bar, it may send your blood sugar for a roller coaster ride. Your blood sugar goes up quickly, causing your pancreas to secrete too much insulin, which causes your blood sugar to drop. That's why you can't stop at one chocolate bar. Eating sweets on an empty stomach causes your blood sugar to rise quickly and then plummet to a lower level coinciding with a feeling of immediate energy followed by a feeling of being very tired.

To help minimise this effect, when you have an urge for sweets and you have an empty stomach, ask yourself if you really want the chocolate bar or if your blood sugar is low because you are hungry. Have something to eat, then if you still want the chocolate bar, have it at that time. Remember that eating sweets and desserts after a meal prevents sugar highs and lows, because on a full stomach it takes longer for the sugar to hit your bloodstream. Continue this process of self-discovery.

It is natural to want sweets when your blood sugar level is low and you are physically hungry. In order for you to remain in charge of the situation try this method of thinking and action.

- Eat regularly to prevent your blood sugar level from dipping too low.

- Eat a balance of carbohydrates and protein to allow a slower release of blood sugar into your bloodstream.

- If you have not eaten for three to four hours, have a more substantial snack such as bread, yogurt, low-fat crackers, or fruit with low-fat cheese, glass of milk, etc.

Promise yourself that if you still want the cake or sweets, you can have them later on. In this way you are not denying yourself. You are understanding your body signals better and helping to distinguish between a craving and a physiological (physical) reason for the craving. You are dealing with the physiological reason first (i.e. low blood sugar). After that the psychological reason may seem less prominent.

CONFRONTATION IS A LIFETIME SKILL

In a confrontation situation dieters would say that you shouldn't have a chocolate bar because it is illegal. It is not on your diet sheet. The fact that it is forbidden causes you to think about it more and want it more. When you confront this urge and don't give in, this act of denial is termed willpower.

If someone is successful in losing weight, the person is said to have more willpower. A better term is 'won't power'. You think that denying the chocolate bar and not responding to the external cue will make it easier to remain in control. Do you really want the sweet or do you think you want it simply because it is there and it is habit? Confronting the urge to eat the sweets will give you the confidence to tune into your natural body signals. Believe in yourself. Listen to your body with regard to physical and psychological hunger. This will help you to distinguish between what you really want versus what you think you want due to habit. Confrontation is meeting the situation head on, and dealing with the cause of the problem. It is a positive skill. Learning to change damaging, self-defeating thoughts that lead to overeating by confronting them is a powerful tool.

What are your reasons for overeating? In order to be in charge, you must deal with the reasons for putting on extra weight. To end the constant struggle of dieting for the rest of your life, deal with the cause and find a permanent cure. Masking the cause only gives you temporary relief. Dealing with the cause, however, may result in uncovering some information about yourself that may cause initial pain.

Let's go back to the scenario with the chocolate bar. Dieters see the chocolate on the table and ask: 'Do I really need it?' or 'Should I really have it?' The non-dieter asks: 'Am I really hungry?' or 'Do I really want it?' Non-diet thinking empowers you to make the choice and puts you in charge.

Dieters are not using a technique; they are using denial to deal with the situation. Non-dieters tune into their hunger signals to check for actual hunger. If the blood sugar is low, non-dieters may choose to have a snack first, knowing that the chocolate bar is available later on. Otherwise, eating chocolate on an empty stomach, when your blood sugar is low, may lower it even further after the initial high. This could cause you to be unable to stop at one chocolate bar.

Eating the cake mixture because you believe that you can't or shouldn't have the cakes is also part of the denial process that occurs with dieting. With our philosophy, you know that you can have the cakes after supper so why eat the cake mixture? The unexpected surprise may be that you feel satisfied with your supper and no longer desire the cakes since you know that you can have them later on if you want to. In other wards, you are not denying yourself, you are allowing yourself to have the cakes. The fact that you can savour them without guilt and enjoy them whenever you want, decreases your desire for them.

Confrontation decreases the incidence of automatic eating, that is, eating simply because it is there. If you do have the cakes after supper, they will have less effect on your blood sugar because it will take longer for the effect of the sugar to reach your bloodstream. And you will probably eat much less.

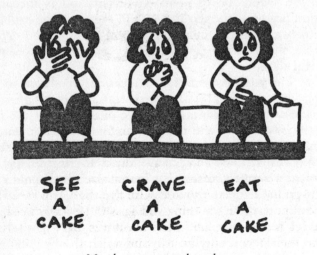

SEE
A
CAKE

CRAVE
A
CAKE

EAT
A
CAKE

Monkey see, monkey do.

Test yourself. When you haven't eaten for a few hours and your blood sugar level is low, walk into a restaurant. You see a nice assortment of cakes that you want. Recognising why you want the cakes is important. First sit down and have a meal.

Taste and savour the meal and you will feel satisfied. The desire for the cake decreases. The waiter comes up to show you the assorted cakes on the dessert tray but do you really want the sweet? Remember, calories are wasted if you are not having what you want, when you want it.

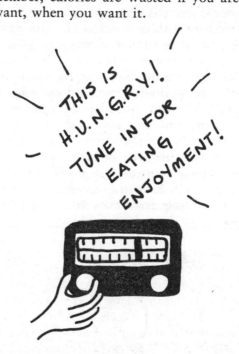

Here's the time to use confrontation. Are you really hungry or just curious to know how it tastes? If you can't resist, try sharing the cake with a friend and practise the confrontation technique to combat automatic eating. Or perhaps recall the many times the dessert looked better than it actually tasted. If you order and can't eat it all, there's nothing wrong with taking the rest home or leaving it on your plate. After all, if it is no longer satisfying to you, then it will only go to your waist.

Dieters react differently. They see the dessert and want it. They may start to eat it simply because of the external cue of sight. Dieters may even choose to eat less food in order to have the dessert. This counting calories could lead to trouble. If dieters don't eat foods with enough substance, the sweet will ultimately create low blood sugar and the craving for sweets will continue. The only gain is a few more pounds. A sense of failure is felt for losing control and cheating on the diet. On the other hand, if the dieter wants the sweet and denies herself physically, this can lead to a binge or preoccupation with the denied food.

Confrontation does not mean total denial. It means that you will be satisfied with a small handful of crisps rather than the whole bag. Confrontation means tuning into your needs at the moment.

Janet baked some great chocolate brownies for Saturday dinner dessert. She wondered what to do with the leftover brownies. Taking them to work or giving them away is the 'out of sight, out of mind' mentality of dieters. Why should she give them away? The rest of the family likes them. Once the new way of thinking is established, the brownies stay in the fridge. But since a small piece satisfies both Janet and her partner, the brownies may get stale. Instead of gobbling them all up, Janet now freezes her baking and takes out a small portion that satisfies everyone.

Confrontation can apply to any aspect of life, not just food. People often eat for other reasons that are not food related. Loneliness, anxiety, depression, anger, stress may be temporarily relieved by food. This is using food as a comforter to make everything seem all right. Accept that it is normal to feel depressed sometimes. If you allow yourself to experience these feelings you may discover why you are distressed and be able to work through the feelings so they won't seem so severe next time.

When you eat for reasons other than physical hunger, you are eating to satisfy your psychological hunger. Your physical hunger may be on 'full' when your psychological hunger is on 'empty'. This means that you are not focusing on the food but using it as a crutch to help you deal with the situation. In this state you can eat a packet of biscuits without even realising what you are doing since you are preoccupied with the psychological problem. To help you get more psychological enjoyment from food, try tasting and savouring it when eating it.

The end result of eating less on this programme may be the same as if you were on a diet. However, the reason for eating less is very different. It's not because you have to. If you taste and savour your food you are likely to be satisfied with less.

If you are not getting psychological enjoyment from the food by tasting and savouring the experience, then you require more food to satisfy you. The problem that caused you to eat in the first place is still there. Confront your problems and deal with them. This will satisfy your inner self and you won't have to eat as a substitute. If you hide your problems, you are not dealing with the inside so the outside will reflect what's going on inside. You can change what you are by changing what goes on in your mind.

If you eat because you are physically tired and are using the food for energy, perhaps you need to go to bed earlier. Otherwise, you are eating to stay awake rather than addressing your real need for sleep. If you are lonely and eat to keep yourself company or for entertainment, maybe you don't value your own company enough. You can be with someone and be lonely or you can be alone and not be lonely. It's all a matter of attitude. As you start to feel better about yourself, you will begin to find interests that keep you occupied and allow you to be constructive. It is worth the effort to make a nice meal for yourself and enjoy it. Falling into the tea-and-toast syndrome when you are alone becomes boring. Because you no longer enjoy or look forward to eating, you may actually end up eating more food, trying to get your psychological satisfaction.

Pamper yourself. You are worth it. Proper nutrition is the fuel for your body. Regular activity helps you to extract more energy to invigorate you in order to reach your potential. Notice your positive qualities. Don't always be down on yourself. Your negative attitude drains your energy. Focus on the positive, and on lifestyle changes. Find the reasons behind your eating, confront them and deal with them. (See Chapter 4 in *Diet breaking* by Mary Evans Young.)

Dieters eat when under stress. Non-dieters do not. Switch your thinking to that of a non-dieter, and you will be less likely to eat under stress. In fact, when dieting, stressful situations cause you to go off your diet. Why does this happen? It happens because dieting in itself puts a stress on your body as well as your mind. Using the principles suggested, stressful situations can be handled with more confidence and authority.

Audrey, a person with diabetes, enrolled in our programme. She related her present health problems to the dieting she had done in the past. She was undergoing very stressful situations at work which would normally cause her to eat and gain weight. To her surprise, when she stepped on the scales, Audrey had lost weight. By not dieting, Audrey was no longer preoccupied with food. She learned to listen to her body and allow her hunger levels to control her food intake naturally, and so can you.

'I can't be on a diet when I'm on holidays. My friend will expect me to eat her home baking.' Does this sound familiar? You're not on a diet now but if your tastes are changing to healthier foods, why do you have to eat those high-fat/high-sugar foods that no longer satisfy you?

Eating to please others can be stressful. It puts the control in the hands of the host or hostess. When you are offered some food, you have a choice to take it or refuse it. If you really want the particular food item, then have it. If you don't want it because you don't particularly care for the food or you aren't hungry, say something such as, 'Thank you, I'm full right now, maybe later.' In this way you are leaving the door open to have the food later when you may actually want it or perhaps you may not want it at all.

Asking for a small piece when the cake is being cut can satisfy your curiosity as well as pleasing your host or hostess while allowing you to practise the principles of the most enjoyment coming from the first and last few bites of whatever you eat. You can always have more if you want it. This also takes a lot of pressure off the hostess who won't feel she has to prepare so much food for her guest.

Do you feel you have to cook lots of food before visitors come in order to make an impression? Remember, true friends and family come to visit because they value your company. Food does not have to be the centre of attraction. When you visit family or friends, reassure them that you have come mainly to see them. They will realise that they do not have to go to as much trouble when you visit. Discuss your change of eating style with your friends. Observe non-dieters in social situations. Food is usually not the centre of attention for them, only a pleasant accent.

If your meal will be later than usual, it's a good idea to have a snack before going out. This will prevent you from feeling famished, which may result in eating quickly without tasting your food, or eating too much.

Distraction is another useful skill that can be used in situations where you have an urge to eat brought on by psychological hunger. Jim was used to finishing his meal every day with dessert. Is this urge for a sweet due to physical hunger or to habit? In his case, it was simply habit. Remembering that urges gradually peak and then disappear, he temporarily distracted himself and the urge went away.

If having a dessert is simply a habit, then distracting yourself for a few minutes after the meal will cause the urge to go away. If there is some other underlying reason for wanting dessert, then it needs to be confronted. Try distracting yourself with an activity that you enjoy that uses your hands, or physically or mentally takes you away from the food situation. This skill is useful in situations where you are trying to break a habit. This form of replacement is only effective on a temporary basis before using confrontation. It can help you to collect your thoughts but it doesn't get to the root cause of the problem.

Doing activities that you enjoy could include going for a walk, having a bubble bath, doing a puzzle, sewing, dancing, listening to classical music, or deep breathing. If the urge for a sweet was due to an external cue such as smelling cakes baked in a bakery, then walking on may allow the urge to go away. The reason this will work is that you distracted yourself for the first few minutes when the urge was at its peak. By distracting yourself at this time, the urge will gradually diminish.

However, if there is a greater underlying cause than the external cues of sight or smell or habit, the urge will recur once the activity is finished. The activity is merely a 'cop-out' from your desire for the food. It's a temporary substitute rather than a skill. You will still have to confront these feelings to minimise the chances of them causing you to eat.

Suppose you had a fight with your spouse that makes you angry enough to want to devour tons of calories to help make you feel better. In this way, you are trying to mask your feelings instead of dealing with them directly. Screaming at your spouse won't solve the problem either, no matter how angry you are. You may decide to go for a walk to allow yourself to calm down, think things over, and plan a strategy for when you come back. This temporary distraction could be helpful in allowing you to think and assess the situation. However, you will still have to confront the situation when you get back. If you don't, out will come the biscuit tin.

Here's a new way of viewing distraction. Ask yourself what's happening in your life that is annoying or painful. Are you avoiding facing it or thinking about it by the distraction of eating?

When you are using distraction techniques, it is important to find an activity that you enjoy. You can acquire a taste for enjoyable activities just as you can acquire a taste for less fattening food. My husband enjoys classical music. By going with the flow, I have learned to appreciate it and use it as a form of distraction to mentally take myself away from the situation or the day's cares.

On the other hand, if you do not enjoy the activity, using it as distraction will not work to alleviate the problem at hand. For example, you might do ironing as a form of distraction even though you do not like ironing. This is using the diet mentality of substituting something inferior rather than finding excitement in a new hobby. You may feel deprived and still turn to food when you are finished. If you are not getting your psychological enjoyment from other activities, then you may turn to food to find that release. Look within and you may discover hidden talents that you would like to explore that can help you fulfil yourself more positively.

In order to confront your hunger and your inner feelings, it is important to understand what 'hunger' feels like. People who have been on so many diets are so out of tune with their bodies that they are no longer able to know what it means to feel hungry. If you are still not in tune with your hunger signals, review Chapter 6. This is the key to helping you succeed. **Remember that anything worth doing is worth doing until you learn to do it well! So practise, practise, practise.**

Diets show you how to ignore your hunger signals. If you are hungry and the diet sheet says not to eat, then you do not eat. You may drink something that temporarily makes you feel satisfied, only to be famished later on. Babies know when they are hungry. Adults ignore the signals because they are influenced by society's obsession with weight. Children too are subjected to parental restraint. Parents don't want their children to be large and this causes restrained eating. Statements such as 'Don't you think you've had enough?' can worry the child and cause secretive eating. A child's or teenager's food needs are much greater than those of an adult. There is the danger that growing bodies will get insufficient calories or nutrients for proper growth. Another danger is instilling the 'diet mentality' into young people.

Dealing with the cause rather than restricting eating is a more positive approach. Reinforce this by putting a family focus on active living, and fill in leisure time with lifestyle activities rather than centring activity around food.

Accept your body shape and that of your child. Unrealistic expectations are the very seedbed of depression. Breaking free of them unleashes the power to break free of the diet mentality.

CLEANING YOUR PLATE – HABIT OR NEED

Back in the days when you were growing up, finishing everything on your plate may have been from necessity. During the Depression, you never knew when or if you were going to get another meal. Eating everything just in case you would have to go hungry for a while was accepted.

This philosophy of wasting nothing may have been passed on to the children of the next generation. How often have you heard, 'Eat everything. The children in Biafra are starving,' or 'I'll give you dessert if you finish your meal.' This condition placed on dessert may have caused you to overeat so that you could have the dessert.

This may have been the beginning of putting you out of tune with your internal body signals. You were responding to external cues, not internal ones. You were moving away from your internal instincts and depending on other people's ideas and reactions. No doubt some parents still rely on this method of getting children to eat everything off their plates.

Today's generation of weight watchers seems to be trying to impose food restrictions on the child out of fear that the child will become large like the parent. This instills feelings of deprivation in the child, which leads to binging. Many children today are out of tune with their bodies and, rather than stuffing themselves, may be undereating to comply with the parents' wishes. This can result in inadequate growth, deficiencies, and insufficient calories, causing cravings and secretive eating. Eating disorders will certainly emerge.

In fact, there is an increase in eating disorders. With teenagers, poor body image and society's view of the 'perfect body', stemming from the 'perfect child with designer clothes', may cause teenagers to inflict periods of starvation on themselves to attain this ideal body image. In pursuit of thinness, their health suffers. Perhaps adults are poor role models because they are never satisfied with their own bodies, and constantly going on and off a diet.

Understanding the reasons why a habit has become entrenched allows this newly found insight to help you find the solution. Use the skill of confrontation to help you break the long-lasting habit. The attitude of 'that's just the way I am' will not allow you to succeed in breaking the habit.

Automatically cleaning your plate after each meal is responding to an ingrained habit. You are not in charge, the chef or waitress is. Eating until you are satisfied, and not exceeding that point, may mean leaving something on your plate. If finishing everything from your plate is simply a habit, then you are not denying yourself if you leave something on your plate. After all, you didn't really want it, you simply ate it because it was there.

Stop partway through your meal to consciously decide if you want more. Putting a 'pause' or 'time out' into your meal may surprise you. You'll find you will be full sooner. Remember, it takes roughly twenty minutes for your stomach to tell your brain that you are full.

Ann commented that she had been taught not to waste food. However, if your body does not want any more food, then the extra food just goes to your waist. Out goes the notch on your belt. You are probably not tasting your food at this point, simply eating because everyone else is feasting, because it's the thing to do, especially at social gatherings. Enjoy the event itself, its surroundings, the people, and the entertainment. These will take the main focus away from food. The food need not be the main reason why you attend the event.

At home, automatic eating occurs more easily when the food is served from bowls. You help yourself and the bowls are left on the table. Second and third helpings may be eaten simply because the food is there and it tastes good, rather than because of physical hunger. Even when you're aware of the situation, it's easy to get caught up in the social event of 'dining' and to continue eating and talking.

Make an attempt to focus on eating while you are eating, and on conversation when you are talking or listening. Tune into your body and ask yourself if you really want any more or if your eyes were bigger than your stomach and you took too much. In that case, try not to eat for the sake of eating. Eat until you feel comfortably full. If you don't want it all, leave the rest for tomorrow, give it to your dog, or throw it out.

Eat for energy, not exhaustion. If you overeat, you feel overly full and tired. Eat until you feel comfortably satisfied. That means not undoing the notch on your belt to make it looser. As you begin to tune into your body, you will be better able to judge how much you really want and there will be less waste. It takes time to reach this point.

When food is served directly on to the plate, the control is taken away from you. You may be given too much and feel obliged to finish it so that you do not hurt anyone's feelings. Don't feel that you have to stuff yourself in order to prove that you like something. 'It's really good but I'm full. Maybe I'll have some later,' works well to notify the cook that your stomach is signalling you to stop eating. If you say 'no' and mean it, people will respect your wishes.

If you serve yourself, you are in control of the quantity and type of food that you want. You can be selective, having more of what you like, and less of what you do not like. The bonus is less hassle all round. Using this method, we can all take responsibility for ourselves. Those who want seconds can choose to get up and get some more. Leaving the food in pots also keeps it hot longer. No need to hurry through the food when you know the second portion will still be hot.

For those of you who are still having trouble leaving something on the plate when you really don't want to eat it, try to leave something small on your plate such as a small scoop of potatoes or a few peas, just to break the cycle of having to eat everything. Keep in mind that the purpose of this exercise is to empower you, put you back in the driver's seat where you are in charge of your body and its needs. Eating past the point of satisfaction just for the sake of cleaning your plate does not allow you to listen to your body. Being aware that you do not have to eat everything on your plate can help you to eat only until you are satisfied.

'So what is wrong with taking a little less and still cleaning my plate?' asked Betty. Nothing, provided you really know at this point what your body needs and you are completely tuned in to those needs. The danger of doing this is that many people decide on what quantity they feel they should be eating according to one of the diets they have been on. Rather than taking what they want and what their body desires, they may choose what they believe their body should have according to previous experiences. As you learn to tune into your signals of hunger and fullness, you will begin to take the amount that will satisfy you. In this case, you may finish everything on your plate.

The other danger is that there will always be social occasions where you may not be in control. Without practising this skill of consciously being aware of when you have had enough to eat, it is the social events that may cause you to overeat. Learning to leave something on your plate may help you to be more conscious of your body's needs.

Practise the skill of leaving something on your plate so that you are prepared for the social event. The ingrained habit of cleaning the plate is difficult to overcome, but it can be done. With time, you will be better able to assess what your body wants rather than eat with your eyes and overfill your plate. You will be in charge.

Observe non-dieters: do they actually eat more food or does it seem that they are eating more because they load up on the carbohydrates (potatoes, rice, pasta, grains, vegetables, bread, etc.)? Non-dieters may also leave more on their plates. For example, I eat what I like until I am satisfied, not until my plate is empty. If I can control what I put on my plate by serving myself, then I take only what I like. However, I do experiment with different kinds of foods and give them a chance to be added to my food repertoire.

You may feel at this time that you are in control and that the practice of consciously leaving something on your plate is no longer necessary. You may leave something on your plate only if you are no longer hungry. This is your goal. The conscious effort of leaving something on your plate is merely to break the habit of constantly finishing everything from your plate and ignoring your true inner hunger signals. Practising the skill will ensure that it becomes second nature more readily.

ACTION POINTS

● Check if you are physically hungry. Ask yourself, 'Why am I eating this?' What's happening in your life that is annoying or painful? Are you avoiding facing it or thinking about it by the distraction of eating, or are you really physically hungry?

● What more do you need to do to make eating a pleasurable experience (e.g. set the table attractively)?

● Discuss your change of eating with friends and family who will support you.

● Encourage a 'serve yourself' system at meal times. This will encourage you to be in charge of the amount of food you eat.

● Eat until you are physically satisfied, not overly full. This may mean leaving something on your plate.

8

How Far Have You Come?

Focus on the internal rewards of energy and wellbeing

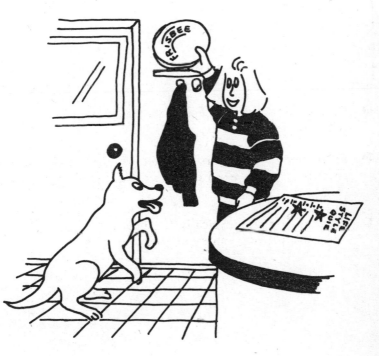

RATING YOUR PROGRESS

In order to apply the principles of this programme successfully and remain focused on this concept, you should step back and assess what lifestyle changes you have made. This gives you an opportunity to see where you have come from, what you have accomplished, and where you are going. It also gives you a chance to set some goals, making you aware of where you can put more time and effort into practising certain skills.

Evaluate your success in functional terms rather than focusing on how many pounds you have lost. Has your quality of life improved? Allow yourself the time to enjoy the process of self-evaluation. An openminded attitude towards these new skills and ideas can help make the breakthrough you need to make the programme work for you. Here is how some clients talk about their lifestyle changes.

'I am eating regularly and no longer starving and binging.'

This is an accomplishment because, as you are now aware, starving and binging can lead to lowering your metabolic rate. Each time you starve, your body compensates by storing more of those calories as fat when you finally do eat. It conserves the calories because your body is afraid that you will starve yourself again.

'I am beginning to understand when and why I'm hungry because I tune in to my natural hunger signals. I know I can eat when I want to, based on my hunger.'

This process of self-discovery allows you to find out why you overate in the first place; it deals with the causes and lets you tune into why you are hungry. This process of self-awareness deals with the causes of eating in a more positive manner.

'I am no longer punishing myself when I eat.'

Eating food without guilt and the act of celebrating food can allow you to taste, savour, and enjoy your food to the fullest. It also allows you to be satisfied with a smaller quantity because you derive not only physical benefit, but psychological satisfaction as well from the food.

'I am eating differently because I want to and it tastes good. I don't get as tired as fast. I am able to complete my housework without sitting down to rest.'

The gradual preference for lower-fat types of foods and increasing activity will build up your endurance so that you feel better and can do more in less time.

'I accept myself the way I am. I like myself.'

Self-acceptance allows you to believe in yourself and your ability to be able to listen to your body with regard to its food and activity needs. It channels your energy so that you can make positive lifestyle changes and gives you the confidence that you need. Otherwise, if you are always negative about yourself, this causes an energy drain where little to nothing is accomplished.

'I'm really thinking how different foods affect my body (metabolic rate and blood sugar). I am eating a balance of carbohydrates and proteins at meals, and feeling more satisfied.'

Cutting calories affects your metabolic rate, causing you to reach a plateau after the initial weight loss. Accept that diets don't work and that rather than cutting calories, the real answer is shifting the type of calories that you take into your body. Eating more carbohydrates gives you the energy to run your body. The balance of protein that is right for you gives you the sustaining energy, stabilising your blood sugar. In this way, you will not have the highs and lows common to diets. This can help to stabilise your mood and general feeling of wellbeing.

By eating more carbohydrates, you are eating more of those calories that burn more energy in the process of their digestion and are less efficient in converting into fat. Simply by eating more carbohydrates you have automatically decreased the total fat content of your meals. By listening to your body, you are allowing your body to determine the energy level that you need on a daily basis. It will be different all the time. Some days you may need more food to make you feel satisfied, and some days you will need less. Some days you may prefer to have a dessert, and other days you will not. Listening to your body's needs and desires will allow you to get the most 'punch' from your meal.

'I've started to alter cooking habits to reduce fat. I am eating more fruit and vegetables, not restricting myself to the non-starchy vegetables.'

As fat content of meals is gradually being decreased, a taste for less fattening foods is being acquired. For example, the comment, 'I now prefer chips prepared in the oven rather than in the deep fryer,' demonstrates this point. Deanna was surprised to notice that after a number of months of gradually cutting back the fat content of her meals, she found fried chicken to be too greasy. She no longer enjoyed this meal and no longer chose to order it. Remember that food choices are built on cultivated preference rather than rigid self-control.

The gradual process of cutting back on your total fat intake in cooking, food choices, and baking is crucial in order to actually change your preference to foods that are lower in fat content.

Going straight from cheddar cheese to cottage cheese is a sudden drop in fat content. It can be a shock to your system causing you to shift back to the higher fat cheese. If you eat cottage cheese simply because it is good for you rather than because you like it, then you are in the diet mentality and your change in eating will not be permanent. In fact, if you can't acquire a taste for the low-fat food, this can prevent you from enjoying your meal, and you may find yourself looking in the cupboards for something that you really enjoy. 'Gradual' implies going from cheddar cheese to low-fat mozzarella cheese, possibly combining the two and eventually going down to low-fat mozzarella cheese. Try other low-fat cheeses such as quark and ricotta, but make them tasty by adding canned fruit in its own juice or some jam.

'I am understanding physical hunger and eating when I am physically hungry.'

Using food to fuel your energy needs feeds the body not the mind. Only then will your clothes begin to get looser.

'I am confronting my psychological hunger.'

This is an important skill not only to deal with hunger and foods but also to help you with all aspects of life so that you can face them in a more positive way. Dealing with the causes of hunger in an assertive manner can reduce the incidence of those feelings.

'I am asking myself if I am really hungry? Do I really want the food?'

This is a form of pausing, where you are confronting yourself to determine your real desires rather than succumbing to eating automatically simply because the food is there. Take the time to check on what you really want.

'I am trying to combat my automatic eating. I'm eating the first few bites and the last few bites and leaving the ones in the middle.'

Becoming aware of your eating, enjoying the act of eating, and eating only what you want allows you to be selective in your eating. Using the above technique can allow you to discover the enjoyment of testing food, noting the quantity that you need to satisfy you.

'I am more aware of when and why I am eating and I am dealing with it in a more positive fashion.'

Getting to know yourself and becoming more conscious of the reasons behind your compulsive eating can allow you to deal with the causes. Once the reasons are resolved, the psychological eating decreases.

'I am beginning to be more active and actually enjoy it.'

Fun and enjoyment are the keys to lifestyle change. A gradual increase in physical activity is important. Your body and mind adapts to the change. You learn to enjoy physical activity, actually missing it when you do without it. Physical activity becomes part of you and your routine. The dieter will say, 'Let's go for a walk to the cake shop. We'll wear off the calories by walking so let's have the cake as our reward for doing the exercise.' The non-dieter will say, 'I went for a walk and I feel great.' The walk becomes the reward in itself. It is an intrinsic reward, coming from within. Action creates motivation. If you wait until you are motivated, action may never take place. External motivation, such as walking to the cake shop for a reward, is only temporary motivation.

'I am more in charge of food.'

By empowering yourself and giving yourself the tools (skills and techniques) to make the choices, you take charge of food and your life. These skills can last a lifetime and be used in any aspect of your life.

REWARDS THAT REALLY WORK

'If you want dessert, you'd better make sure that you eat everything on your plate, Ellen.' The mother who says this makes the dessert the reward for a job well done, whether it was finishing your plate of food or transferring the food reward idea to other tasks such as doing your homework, etc. Why couldn't the act of eating or accomplishing something be the internal reward in itself? Why do we always feel that we need an external reward to finish the task or finalise the moment? Enjoy the meal itself and if you want dessert, have it, but not because it is your reward for finishing the meal. Revel in your accomplishments and experience the feeling of exhilaration without needing food to provide the finishing touch.

Paul comes home from school and practises his guitar. When he is finished, he goes to watch television as a reward. Why can't the enjoyment extracted from playing the guitar be the immediate reward? This is a healthier way of thinking that will instill positive lifetime habits. Enjoy the new skills that you are learning; focus on the intrinsic reward of the moment.

In the past, rewards may have been essential to keep you on track with your diet. Starving yourself before you weighed in at your diet class resulted in a weight loss that you rewarded by some type of food after the weigh-in. After all, you have been faithful in depriving yourself. And because you are so hungry, something high in fat such as a doughnut is tempting. So off to the cake shop you go.

You equated the result with the weight loss and the natural reward is the thing you have been doing without – food. Are you really making a lifestyle change? No! What you are doing is only temporary, a means to an end. You may constantly repeat this cycle over and over again. Losing the weight, resuming old eating habits, regaining the weight, another diet. Your sense of wellbeing and self-esteem goes down as your weight goes up, and you have a feeling of powerlessness.

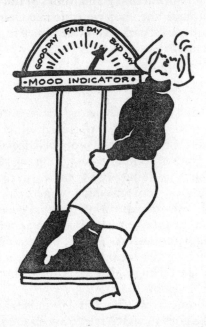

Realise that you count by allowing the way you feel about yourself and your improved health to be your reward. This internal reward is more likely to last. A positive feeling in itself allows you to keep on the road to lifestyle changes. Look at your accomplishments and remember that lapses from time to time are part of progress.

Unrealistic expectations can cause depression about your weight. The weight you lose should not be the goal or the focus of your actions. Rather, improvement in health is the key to your long-term success. Applying some of the skills and techniques you are learning will allow you to experience mini-successes and reduce the number of setbacks that occur. Focus on these gradual changes. They are progress and they can help keep your goals realistic and in focus.

Attempt to normalise your eating habits. The scale doesn't rule your life and should not be ruling how you feel each day. Take a look inside yourself for the clues. Soon the outside will begin to reflect your renewed confidence. You may be walking straighter, taller. You'll be in charge.

Never mind what others say and think. Jealousy because you are in charge of your food and your life may cause others to try to sabotage your best efforts. Don't be fooled into thinking that another diet will get the weight off faster. Quick weight loss results in quick weight gain.

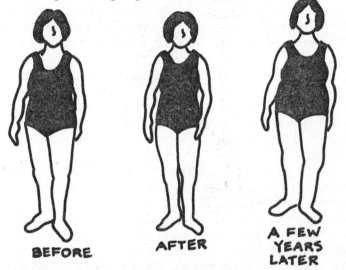

BEFORE   AFTER   A FEW YEARS LATER

Start living for the present instead of always focusing on the future. Enjoy and savour the moment. The more psychological benefit that you can extract from life, the less you will need food to fill this void and the greater will be your inner rewards. Being desperate for weight loss prevents it from happening naturally. Focusing on lifestyle changes allows you to master new ways of thinking. Practice will allow you to internalise them.

As lifestyle changes become second nature, you will feel more energetic and confident that you are able to steer your life on to a path of health and vigour. With time your body will adjust naturally to the weight that you were predetermined to be. Keep in mind that these outward effects will happen more quickly only in those who allow it to happen naturally. Forcing makes these changes temporary. It doesn't allow you to 'feel' and 'experience' them. Lifestyle changes require effort to become established. Practice makes them easier.

Diets are initially easy because you operate within a prescribed regime. However, they soon become boring and monotonous. Lifestyle changes require a change in thinking that motivates you. If you enjoy the process and heed the lifetime skills, time will not be a factor. Stress the positive, go with the flow, allow it to happen. It is a self-fulfilling prophecy. Believe in yourself, and have the confidence that you can make those changes. You will be successful because you have learned from past failures and allowed yourself to grow. You will move forward.

We all operate on a conscious or unconscious reward system. The most effective rewards are the ones you reap from your own individual value system. The achievement of meeting your own standard is a euphoric experience. Your own opinion about yourself is what counts; the opinions of others are not as important.

If you live for others' comments and compliments, consider what happens after you have lost weight. The praise, encouragement, and compliments will stop after people have become accustomed to your new physical appearance. Will you then feel there is no more purpose in trying to keep the weight off? Or will you put the weight back on to gain attention? Or maybe you have realised that changing the outside self alone does not make you instantly happy or allow your problems to disappear. You are still the same person, the same individual. Your attitude or the way you think, feel, or act towards yourself or others has not changed. Your attitude towards food or life has not changed. It remains the same and so you will set yourself up for gaining the weight back.

Work on discovering yourself and what makes you eat. Deal with the causes and forces, and allow yourself to develop skills to improve your inner self. These can channel your energies into being the best that you can be! The inner strength that you gain will begin to reflect outwards.

REVIEW YOUR PROGRESS

- Am I eating regularly and no longer starving and binging?

- Am I beginning to understand when and why I am hungry and actually starting to tune in to my hunger signals?

- By gradually decreasing fat content over the past few weeks, am I beginning to acquire a taste for less fattening foods?

- Am I eating a balance of carbohydrates and proteins at meals, putting more emphasis on increasing the carbohydrate content without feeling guilty?

- Am I enjoying the full experience of eating and am I eating until I feel satisfied in order to fuel my energy needs rather than my psychological needs?

- Am I tuning in to how I feel and how my body feels, no longer relying on the scales to determine how my day will go?

- Am I feeling more energetic and more content with myself?

- Am I starting to use skills to combat automatic eating and confrontation to deal with those urges that make me want to eat even though I am physically satisfied?

- Am I beginning to participate in more physical activity and actually enjoying it?

- Am I more aware of what I am eating?

AFFIRMATIONS TO MOVE YOU FORWARD

Use the following phrases as affirmations to be repeated frequently. They will help you to set your mind on to a positive track.

- I like myself. I feel good about myself. I'm a worthwhile person no matter what anybody says or does. I'm going to have a great day.

- I believe in myself and have the confidence that I can listen to my body. I know what to eat and when my body is hungry. I know the level of activity that is suited to me to allow physical activity to give me energy, not exhaustion.

- When I feel like eating as a result of feelings, I will first stop, meet the situation head-on, and attempt to deal with the reason for my eating. I will work at preventing the reason from happening again. I will look at ways of dealing with these feelings in those cases where the cause cannot be prevented or eliminated.

- I realise that eating only until I am satisfied may mean leaving something on my plate. In order for me to break the automatic habit of finishing everything on my plate, I will give myself permission to eat only until I am satisfied, and not feel compelled to eat all the food on my plate, even if it means leaving something.

Use the above affirmations regularly to help more you forward on the road to healthy living.

ACTION POINTS

● Evaluate your successes in function terms rather than focusing on how many pounds you have lost. Acknowledge (in your journal if you have one) your practical achievements.

● Continue to differentiate between your feelings of physical versus psychological hunger.

● Start developing strategies to meet your psychological needs. You may have a range of needs which will vary in complexity and difficulty, and in the amount of work required to resolve them. Start identifying useful resources outside this book that may help, such as friends, books, organisations, workshops, counselling.

● Start to address automatic eating by concentrating on what you eat and dealing with why you eat.

● Allow improved health and positive feelings about yourself to be your real rewards.

● Remember to do the positive affirmations regularly.

9

Maximum Satisfaction from Food

Use skills of confrontation to cope with bursts of psychological hunger. Stop: taste, savour, and enjoy your food to the fullest.

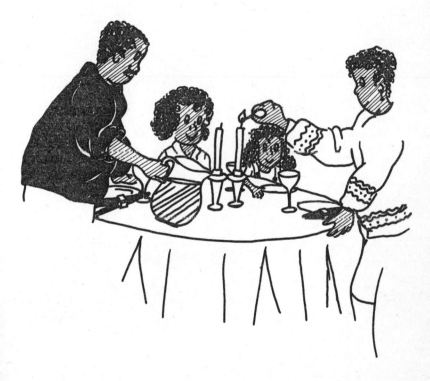

If you are eating only to feed your psychological hunger, then these calories are wasted. Take the time to taste and savour your food and you'll notice that you will actually be satisfied with less. Why? Because you took the time to satisfy your psychological hunger from the food.

FOCUS ON FOOD – PAYING ATTENTION

When you don't pay attention to what you are eating, you literally cheat yourself from getting satisfaction and pleasure from the food. Then, in searching for the sense of wellbeing that you denied yourself, you eat more than you need or want. Perhaps the tendency to avoid paying full attention when you are eating comes from the belief that you don't deserve to be good to yourself. If you actually sit down and enjoy your food, you have to acknowledge that you're giving something to yourself. This is very difficult for many people to do – especially women. Also, many people pride themselves on being able to do several things at once. They say, 'I work all the time; in fact, I don't even take time off for lunch.' They think it's efficient to eat while they are doing ten other things, rather than wasting time on eating without doing anything else. Do these people really taste their food or are they eating it only because it's there?

Experience the different taste sensations, textures, and aromas. The outcome of not tasting your food can be:

- eating more food to satisfy your cravings;

- overeating due to unconscious eating and being out of tune with your body; or

- nibbling throughout the evening because you don't remember eating anything.

Any bite of food that goes into your mouth deserves attention. When you eat, do nothing but eat. Even if you're eating only a handful of raisins, sit down, take a deep breath, relax, and focus on the raisins. If you are doing anything else while you are eating, you are not concentrating on the subtleties of the tastes and flavours of the food. In this way, you not only deprive yourself of the enjoyment of the food, but you may form an association between eating and some other activity (see Chapter 12).

When you are eating by yourself it is easy to pay attention only to your food. When you are with another person it is more difficult to concentrate only on your food. Here's a tip. When eating with others, spend about thirty seconds focused on your food, then put your fork down and focus your attention on the other person and the conversation. You cheat the person you're with if you eat while conversing, and you deprive yourself of the pleasure of the food if you talk while eating. So, alternate eating and talking. This will allow you to receive optimum pleasure from the food and your relationships.

Other Frames of Mind that Can Lead to Absent-minded Eating

THE JUGGLER
You're a person who always juggles twenty things at a time, and one of the twenty is eating. Have you finished all the kids' lunch leftovers during the half hour you spent putting away the laundry and listening to your neighbour on the telephone?

These people often feel that taking time out to eat is not productive. Yet focusing on eating allows you to put the 'pause' into your day and gives your stomach time to signal to your brain that you are full. The result is that it translates to decreased nibbling and increased energy and productivity later on.

THE ABSENTEE OWNER
These lost souls are dreamy, unconscious eaters who don't even notice they're eating. While they're licking an ice cream cone, they're also day-dreaming, reading, shopping, or watching television. Suddenly, they realise with a shock that the ice cream cone has mysteriously disappeared.

THE GIVER
Givers try to be all things to all people and to perform many functions at a time. These people, often mothers, spread themselves too thin in their workloads, while their waistlines, not so ironically, often become considerably thicker. They telephone committee members, wash dishes, referee family squabbles, cook dinner, and write a report for work while at the same time picking away at food.

Make it a routine to eat only when you are sitting. There is no joy in eating on the run. Such eating is not satisfying and it encourages nibbling. It's interesting how, when you eat on the run, the mind erases the meal but the body doesn't. If you sit down at the table every time you eat, you will naturally pay more attention to your food. You will then enjoy conscious eating and you will remember what you ate.

THE TIME TRAVELLER
To get the most satisfaction from your food, your focus must be in the present. Time travellers either dwell in the past (feeling guilty about what they've done) or the future (worrying about bad things before they happen). John Curtis, founder and director of the University of Wisconsin Stress Management Institute, believes that ninety percent of stress is brought on by not living in the present moment and worrying about what's already happened, what's going to happen, or what could happen.

Accept responsibility for the past, face the future with confidence, and focus on today, learning to taste, savour, and enjoy. It seems obvious, doesn't it, to taste and enjoy each bite? Why then is it so rarely practised? Experiment with this theory. Try eating the same breakfast (one day in a hurry and the next day relaxed) at the table and actually tasting the food. Do you notice a difference in how long it keeps you satisfied?

Eating on the run or while focusing on what you have to do next rather than on the moment at hand deprives you of the psychological pleasure of the present. Constantly living for the future deprives you of the enjoyment of what is going on now. Take the time to savour the enjoyment of discovering your inner being as you begin to realise that you are important enough to pamper yourself with the time to taste and savour your meal. After all, you count!

George came to the YCCD group one day and told us that he had had second helpings because the food tasted so good. On further probing, he said that he had rushed to get to the group and had hurried through his meal. He pointed out that normally he would have been amply satisfied with the first helping. Make sure you try this exercise. It will give you new insight into the true meaning of tasting and savouring your food.

It is important to ensure that you are eating the foods that you love. There are no good foods or bad foods, no 'dos' or 'don'ts'. You can eat anything your body loves to eat. Listen to your body. At first you may hear your body say it wants all those 'forbidden' foods you never allowed yourself when you were dieting. But as long as you eat only when you're hungry and stop when you're full, your body will soon crave the foods that it needs for your health and wellbeing. Care enough to listen. Be creative. Savour all the flavours of your food and drink, and when you eat, enjoy the food without washing it down with liquids.

VARIETY IS THE SPICE OF LIFE

Ann felt that she was doomed to suffer on a medically pre-scribed low-fat diet. She ate the same thing every day for breakfast and lunch. There was a little more variety in her dinners but there was certainly no surprise or anything out of the ordinary to perk up her taste buds. She was bored, bored, bored with her food plan. No wonder she was prone to nibbling and feelings of deprivation.

It is so important to have something different to eat that is enjoyable so that your mind and attention are drawn back to the eating experience. New recipes, a variety of different breads and cereals, brightly coloured vegetables, a new way of presenting an old favourite meal, or any number of other 'attention grabbers' can be used so that they will register psychologically and you will know you have eaten.

Presentation of the meal can add to the enjoyment. It's fun emphasising different colours and textures. Try not to fall into the winter trap of humdrum vegetables and fruits that are far from exciting when you see them over and over again. Carrots, apples, and oranges are great, but if you don't think of different ways to serve them they become monotonous.

When the fancier vegetables and fruits are out of season they are more expensive. But if you are unsatisfied with the meal due to its lack of 'oomph' you will follow it by a rich dessert or chocolate bar to satisfy your psychological craving.

Switching over to our way of eating may involve eating a greater proportion of vegetables and fruits that are more costly when out of season. However, clients tell me that overall, their food bills are less because of their lower consumption of convenience foods. Finding more satisfaction from the regular meal reduces the tendency to want more later on. Compare the difference for yourself and you may be pleasantly surprised!

LEARNING TO TASTE, SAVOUR AND ENJOY

Eating slowly can maximise your enjoyment of food and provide an earlier feeling of fullness for a given quantity of food consumed. It will also slow down the release of sugar into the bloodstream. Eating quickly can minimise your enjoyment of food and fool your body's appetite control mechanism into wanting more.

Listening to classical music while you eat may decrease your appetite and benefit digestion. A recent study performed by the Health and Stress Clinic at Johns Hopkins University shows that people who listened to classical music while eating took longer to finish the meal, took fewer bites per minute, and were satisfied with one helping. Those who listened to rock music and marching tunes ate faster, ate more per forkful, and asked for second helpings.[1]

Is filling up on water before a meal the answer? You will feel bloated and will not be able to eat as much. Is this dealing with your physical hunger or temporarily trying to avoid it? Will it not lead to greater hunger later on?

Does focusing on your eating mean putting your fork down between bites? Think about it. Isn't this an external cue? It may work for a while, but it's not natural and may be difficult to internalise as a new way of eating.

TECHNIQUES TO INTERRUPT AUTOMATIC EATING

- Create a relaxed atmosphere prior to eating so that the mood is set to enjoy the meal. Soothing music in the background may help create the mood. Dine, don't simply eat.

- Focus on what you are eating (taste, flavour, texture, and aroma) while you are eating. Don't smother your food with too many condiments that can mask the flavour. As you gradually cut back on the fats and enhance the flavour with herbs and spices, you will begin to enjoy the natural flavour of food.

- Build in a 'pause' partway through your meal. Pause during your meal: start with thirty seconds. Gradually increase time to one, two, and three minutes. Initially, this may be a conscious effort to interrupt the process of automatic eating. This 'pause' will help to put you in touch with your feelings of hunger and fullness.

- Focus on the food and the eating of it while you are eating. When you are talking to others, put your fork down and focus on the conversation. Otherwise, you end up talking with your mouth full of food and deprive yourself of the true enjoyment of either activity. Practising this technique is more natural than the artificial method of putting your fork down between bites.

- Come to the meal pleasantly hungry, but not famished. This will help to regulate your speed of eating. Build in snacks if you anticipate that your meal is going to be delayed.

- Be less efficient when eating. For example, when you are having a soup or salad and sandwich, don't be so organised that you eat the soup while holding the sandwich in the other hand. Then you will finish the meal in no time. Instead try making the soup piping hot and finish it before starting the sandwich. Then you are fully enjoying the soup and extending the time frame of your meal. Or eat a salad prior to the meal. Its texture will get you into the habit of chewing food more and will help to slow you down. After all, it's your special time. Enjoy it!

- Focus on the attitude that goes along with eating slowly rather than simply the behaviour. In other words, if you sit down for a few minutes when you get home, it gives you a chance to break the 'rush-rush' momentum that might have been built up all day. It allows you a chance to reflect on the day's activities. Plan for the meal, and maybe include a snack before dinner to avoid nibbling everything in sight. When you are pleasantly hungry it creates the right mood to help you eat more slowly and naturally.

Naturally slow eaters do not put their forks down between bites. Start observing slow eaters. They are often slimmer but not because of dieting. Non-dieters naturally focus on eating, while they are eating. On the other hand, while talking, they may put their forks down and focus on the conversation. For them eating is not automatic, it is conscious and they are tasting every morsel and enjoying their food.

In order to slow your eating rate, be patient and practise the following techniques until the old patterns are replaced by new ones. The purpose of these techniques is:

- to interrupt the process of automatic eating;

- to give your stomach a chance to register to your brain that you are full; and

- to slow down the release of sugar into the bloodstream.

These methods and techniques can put you on the road to slower eating.

VISUALISATION: MAKING IT HAPPEN

Eating slowly is not simply a change in behaviour; it's a state of mind that in turn will motivate you to fully experience on a regular basis the tastes, textures, aromas, and flavours of dining. Visualising or imagining yourself as being relaxed before you begin the meal, and tasting and savouring your food as you eat will help. Stop at times, put your fork down, and engage in conversation. Your speed of eating will slow down more readily.

To demonstrate how effective this technique can be, recite the following scenario to yourself while soft music is playing in the background. This creates a relaxed atmosphere.

'I have just come home from work. I do some deep breathing and a few stretches for a couple of minutes. Feeling relaxed but hungry, I go to the fridge, get myself a snack (i.e. crackers and milk or whatever I find to be appropriate as a snack). I sit down at the table and enjoy the snack. I get up after five or ten minutes, prepare the meal, and feel less anxious at mealtime. I am able to enjoy the meal and actually feel less hurried. My appetite is pleasantly stimulated for this meal. I'm glad I stopped to have a snack before I ate dinner. Now I can taste and enjoy the food. I am enjoying talking to my family. I stop eating at times to talk to my family about some of the pleasant events of the day's activities. I find myself tasting my food so I am eating more slowly. I realise that whenever I'm hungry, I can get myself something to eat so there is no need to clean off everything on my plate. I am satisfied now. I leave the table feeling satisfied, but not overly full.'

Now close your eyes and picture yourself eating in this manner. Visualise it. See yourself as this new person in charge of your eating, simply because you are enjoying the food, the moment, the company, and the event. Do this at least once a day until it begins to happen naturally and what you visualise becomes reality. No matter what the occasion you will find a way to enjoy it. Your fork still goes down once in a while which puts the 'pause' in your eating, allowing you to decide if you really want more. It breaks the automatic eating and gives you a chance to feel if you are still hungry or are simply eating because the food is there.

Eating quickly may result from allowing yourself to get too hungry. Or you may eat too quickly to prevent the food from getting cold. Think about it. Are you actually allowing yourself to taste and savour the food when you eat quickly? Eating the food more slowly, even if it is cooler, allows you to extract more flavour and tune into the texture and get the enjoyment from the experience of eating. You are learning to view food in a different way.

If you are still concerned that this slower way of eating will allow your food to get cold, try heating the plates beforehand. Some people put them in the heat cycle in the dishwasher or in the oven on low heat. Actually, I find the food still tastes great even though it may be lukewarm. The flavours are more pronounced at this temperature. The extremes of temperature, whether very cold or very hot, do not allow you to experience the most flavour.

This total enjoyment of the food and the event will eventually allow you to be satisfied with less to eat. The end result of eating smaller portions may be the same as diet programmes but the reason for arriving there is different. It is now your choice. Learning, practising, and enjoying add up to health benefits. You have different preferences which help regulate your feeling of fullness. You eat less for different reasons. You are in charge and you make the choices. The valuable skill of visualisation can be used with any type of activity or change that you would like to implement more quickly into your lifestyle. Athletes often use it prior to a big event, when they focus on their style to gain poise and concentration.

You can imagine yourself more active. For example, if you close your eyes and see yourself walking and enjoying it, then you are more apt to want to walk. In this way, you have instilled a positive message in your mind about walking.

When trying this method to help internalise different skills or gain confidence, focus on the action involved. Imagine yourself being positive and making the lifestyle changes that will help you achieve a healthier body rather than focusing on looking thin or seeing yourself as slim. Focus on the enjoyment of the process, not the end result.

REASONS FOR LOSING CONTROL OVER FOOD

As long as you continue to avoid your favourite foods (ones that may be high in calories or high-fat) without confronting the reasons behind your continued cravings, you will continue to deprive yourself psychologically. This sets you up for binging on these foods when you are finally exposed to them.

You want to eat but it isn't because you are physically hungry. You are upset and haven't confronted the situation. You are afraid to confront it so you continue to eat to make yourself feel better temporarily. Feelings of anger, frustration, or loneliness seem to be relieved through eating. However, you are still faced with the situation at hand.

If you continue to ignore your problem or deal with it in an ineffective manner, you will never resolve it and this cycle of eating may lead to gaining more weight. This will further lower your self-esteem. You won't have a good feeling about yourself and you will never be able to take control of the problem and of the food.

During your childhood you may have learned to keep your emotions to yourself. Pent-up feelings of anger can be very bad for your health. Displaying anger in a negative way is called aggression. Displaying anger in a positive, controlled manner is confrontation, which is a form of assertiveness.

Initially, you may want to use distraction to relieve some of your anger. Try going for a walk or going away from the situation to give yourself a chance to gain perspective. This may give you the opportunity to sort things out and better understand what is really troubling you and what you really want to say.

Think before you talk; otherwise, you may say things in anger that you do not really mean. Voicing your feelings in a constructive way can set you free from those pent-up emotions and keep you from feeling the need to eat, to fill this emotional void with food. State your request or your complaint clearly and in a positive manner. Think it through and deal with the situation rationally. You will never know the outcome unless you try to deal with the problem. Spouses or friends cannot read your mind.

It is essential to go back and discover the reasons for your eating and the reasons why you are eating compulsively. Treating your overeating by going on a diet is only a temporary solution. Awareness of the reasons for your overeating is the first step to permanent success.

Congratulate yourself for every success and every new awareness. Change is stressful, so introduce changes gradually, taking it one step at a time. If you introduce just one new lifestyle change this week and repeat it at every opportunity, it will take root and you will take a major step forward. Your aim is to make one small and concrete change and to really enjoy the way it makes you feel. You can derive much satisfaction from the awareness that you are on the right path, one that you alone have chosen to take.

This awareness can lead to action. It allows you to continue to practise the skill of confrontation with regard to the situations themselves, not only with food. After all, it may be the situations that are causing you to eat. If you can make the effort to deal with them, the need for food as a crutch or comforter will no longer be necessary. It will be much easier to eat only when you are actually physically hungry.

Compulsive behaviour can be expressed in many ways. The workaholic has compulsive behaviour that is accepted by society. Yet it can endanger health by putting both physical and mental stress on the body. The resulting burnout affects eating and activity habits. The person becomes stressed out and may compensate by eating too much.

EXAMPLES TO HELP YOU WORK THROUGH YOUR NEW SKILLS AND HELP YOU DISTINGUISH PHYSICAL FROM PSYCHOLOGICAL HUNGER

Example 1

Jane walks by a bakery, smells croissants and wants to have one. This is an example of psychological hunger where Jane is responding to an external cue. She smells it, she wants it. Does she really want it because of hunger or is she just used to responding to the external cue?

What kind of learned skills can she use? An urge to eat builds gradually like a wave, peaks, and gradually reduces. If Jane keeps on walking, the urge may go away if it was elicited simply by the smell of the croissants and she wasn't physically hungry.

If there is a psychological reason for feeling hungry, she may try to confront the urge. If, as Jane keeps walking, she still desires the croissant, there may be another reason for wanting it.. She could find out the reason and deal with it using confrontation skills.

If Jane walks into the bakery and really wants a croissant because it is her favourite snack, should she have one? Yes. If she doesn't, she may think about it for the rest of the day, then raid the fridge when she gets home because she feels deprived.

Jane orders the croissant she wants. She is selective and orders only what she wants. She remembers that most of the satisfaction comes from the first and last few bites of what she is eating. So she tastes and savours the croissant but notices that it doesn't taste as good as it did in her mind. She packs up the rest for her dog. Her other option is to leave whatever is left once she has satisfied her urge.

On the other hand, if Jane was really hungry, a croissant may not be the best choice. They are high in fat and sugar which may send her blood sugar for a roller coaster ride, especially on an empty stomach. And what about all that fat that will just go to body fat? She could try not to let herself get too hungry.

Example 2

It's four o'clock and you are usually hungry at this time. What type of hunger is this? It may be either physical or psychological.

What kind of learned skills can you use? If you haven't eaten for about four hours you are simply physically hungry. In that case, have a snack. If you try to hold off until supper, you may end up famished by that time. This is no way to go to a meal. It does not allow you the opportunity to taste and savour your food.

However, if you had a snack at three o'clock, but you always come home from work hungry, this may be caused by the let down of the day, by loneliness, or habit. You are the only one who can determine what kind of hunger it is and use the appropriate skills to handle it. Confront the urge and deal with the cause.

Check with yourself on the role that food plays for you and your family at different times of the day. Do your children need a snack before supper? Are you concerned about them spoiling their supper, so they remain hungry and cranky until supper time? The idea of a snack is simply to dampen hunger, not to spoil the next meal. Arrive at the table pleasantly hungry, not starved.

You are working against your body when:

- You ignore your natural hunger signals and undereat at the expense of health.

- You overeat to find emotional satisfaction from food rather than from other parts of your life.

- You undereat to try to change your body shape to what you feel is accepted by society.

- You overeat because you are not paying attention to food to derive both physical and psychological satisfaction from it.

Learn to work with your body. Tune into the enjoyment of your life in balance. Meet the situation head on, and delight in your progress.

ACTION POINTS

● Put into practice techniques to interrupt automatic eating (see p208).

● At parties, celebrations, family gatherings etc., concentrate on the event rather than the food.

● Take charge of your food by becoming more self-aware.

Confront the reasons behind your cravings.

Stop, taste, savour and enjoy your food to the fullest. Pay attention to the food you are eating. Be careful not to focus on what you should be doing instead of enjoying the eating experience itself.

Face feelings of anger, frustration, boredom, loneliness.

Learn to be assertive – it is natural to have feelings so don't keep them pent up or attempt to 'eat them away'.

Acknowledge when you have a problem and try to deal wit it appropriately, seeking professional help if necessary.

● Practice visualisation, a powerful skill.

See yourself eating slowly in a relaxed fashion.

See yourself enjoying more physical activity.

10

Reading What It's All About

Exercise your choice in the purchase of products
suited to your new tastes

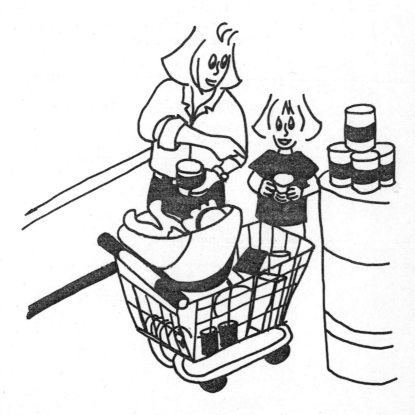

Now it's time to learn how to make the best use of food labels so that you are able to exercise your choice in the purchase of products suited to your new taste for food. The food label is the manufacturer's way of communicating with the consumer. In order to best utilise this handy tool, it is important to understand how to read the label so that you get the information you need to make your decisions.

A BLUEPRINT FOR LABEL READING

The ingredients on the label are listed according to the proportion by weight of the ingredients in the product. The main ingredient in a recipe is first on the list. Check the list for the first five ingredients. If any of them is a source of fat or sugar, then the product is probably high in calories.

Reading only the front of the label can be confusing and even misleading. Take the example of the sugarless chocolate bar. The information on the front of the chocolate bar label makes it sound enticing to the person with diabetes and maybe even to those who are concerned about sugar or weight. It is important to note that the words 'sugarless milk' are on the front of the label in large print while the message to the person with diabetes is in small print and hardly noticeable. The chocolate bar was bought at a store where the owner had a large sign advertising the fact that the chocolate bar was sugarless.

The small print on the back of the label is more revealing. The ingredients are listed as cocoa butter, sorbitol, milk, mannitol, cocoa, ground hazelnuts, skimmed milk, emulsifier, saccharin, vanillin.

The main ingredient is cocoa butter, a fat that will convert into fat in your body very efficiently. Further reading reveals that the bar contains eighty calories. You need to read it carefully, in order to realise that it means eighty calories per serving size of four squares and not eighty calories for the large chocolate bar. With six servings per bar, this equals 480 calories per bar. Most of the calories come from fat. Why does the chocolate bar have so much fat (fifty-six percent of the calories come from fat)? One of the functions of sugar is as a tenderiser. Taking out the sugar requires the addition of fat to bring back that smooth texture. With more sugar, the quantity of fat could be reduced.

Since this product does not contain any granulated sugar necessary for the smooth texture that is part of a good quality chocolate bar, does that mean that it does not contain any sugar at all? The answer is no. Sorbitol and mannitol are sugar alcohols that eventually break down into sugar in your system. Saccharin is an artificial sweetener. Combining these three sweeteners may simulate the taste of sugar but they do nothing for the texture. More fat is needed. The result is a chocolate bar that would not satisfy the chocolate connoisseur. Yet it contains the same number of calories (maybe more) as your old reliable chocolate bar!

The moral here is that if you really want a chocolate bar, don't settle for a substitute that leaves you wanting the real thing. Acquiring a taste for less sugary and fattening foods requires gradual changes, not sudden disappointments. Inferior substitutions can lead to feelings of deprivation, eventually leading to binging on the real food.

Tasting, savouring, and enjoying your real chocolate bar may allow you to be satisfied with less than the whole bar. After all, if you know that you can eat it without guilt and enjoy it and have it at any time, you may eat only what you really want at the time. As you begin to think more like a non-dieter, you may become more selective in the type of chocolate bar you like (i.e. not as sweet due to a taste for less sugary foods).

FACTS ABOUT HEALTH FOODS REVEALED

Many foods lead you to think they are nourishing, but they are not. Don't be lulled into a false sense of security by a healthy-sounding name. Always read labels. Some foods pretend to be health foods but are they really healthy?

Frozen Vegetarian Pasta Even though pasta on its own is fat free, prepared pasta products that omit meat may contain full-fat cheeses that are high in fat. A 10.5-ounce (298-g) serving of one popular frozen vegetable lasagna contains only 225 calories; however, fifty percent of those calories come from the 12.5 grams of fat, which is largely saturated. The dish contains three cheeses and has a breadcrumb topping moistened with partially hydrogenated oils. In contrast, the percentage of fat calories in one regular meat lasagna, another frozen dinner, is only thirty-two percent.

Packaged Pasta Salad Packed in the same way as instant soups, you boil up dried pasta and dehydrated vegetables from one packet. Another packet contains seasonings (including lots of sodium) which you blend with oil for a dressing. Unfortunately, thirty-eight percent of the 190 calories in a 1/2 cup (125 ml) serving of one well-known brand of pasta salad come from eight grams of fat (seven of which you added yourself). *Question whether adding all this fat is necessary.* Another option would be to cook your own pasta (just as quick) and add your own mix of any of the following seasonings by itself or combined with low-fat yogurt: unsalted herbs, Dijon mustard, chili powder, Worcester sauce.

Bran Muffins If the muffins contain bran, they will certainly contain fibre, but it may be very little. Most shop-bought muffins have far more hydrogenated oils, sugar, and eggs in them than oat or wheat bran. Check the ingredients list. If bran is close to the bottom, you're being deceived. Look for whole wheat flour as the main ingredient, not wheat flour (refined white flour).

Carrot Cake If it is dense and moist this indicates a high-fat content. A typical cake may contain more than a cup (250 ml) of oil which has nearly 2000 calories by itself (about 200 calories per slice before adding the other ingredients). *Note* These are all fat calories. Nearly all shop-bought carrot cakes also contain a variety of sugars, refined flour, eggs, and shortening, plus cream cheese and more sugar in the icing. From the health point of view, you'll almost always be better off with apple pie, even though it may be loaded with sugar (this does not apply to people with diabetes).

Banana Cake and Banana Bread These are not much different than chocolate cake. One widely sold banana cake begins with sugar, continues with partially hydrogenated vegetable shortening and then flour. After that comes the bananas. Just as carrot cakes do, banana cakes usually get forty to fifty percent of their calories from fat. Shop-bought banana breads may be as full of fat as the banana cakes. To avoid this, make sure that flour is first on the ingredients list and shortening towards the bottom. Less fat and sugar are required in making your own banana bread.

Frozen Tofu Desserts These are widely advertised as healthy substitutes for ice cream. They are cholesterol- and lactose-free but their calorie and fat content may actually be higher than that of ice cream. *Note* They may also be nearly tofu-free. Half the 230 calories in a four-ounce (113-g) serving of one popular frozen tofu product comes from sugars (high-fructose corn sweeteners, corn syrup, and honey) and the other half from fat (partially hydrogenated). Tofu is ranked fifth on the ingredients list. If the dessert has a chocolate or carob coating this will add more fat and calories.

Popcorn This is a no-fat, low-calorie snack when popped with little or no oil or salt and left unbuttered. *Note* A hot-air popper requires no oil. Microwave popcorn and pre-popped corn usually contain twice as many calories as conventional popcorn, a hefty dose of salt, and more fat per ounce or gram than most biscuits. The fat comes from vegetable oils that are usually hydrogenated (saturated) and sometimes cheese is added as well.

Vegetarian Pâté Some of these pâtés mimic the fatty texture of traditional liver pâté by the addition of fat. One brand lists palm kernel oil (more highly saturated than animal fat) second among its ingredients after water. Peanut oil is listed a little further down the list. *Note* In this case the predominant vegetable ingredient is potato starch.[1]

Peanut Butter Most commercial brands of peanut butter contain salt and sugar, hydrogenated oil (which keeps it from separating), as well as salt and sugar. The kind made solely from peanuts has about fifteen percent less fat and almost no salt. Even though this peanut butter that is made straight from peanuts derives nearly eighty percent of its calories from fat, the fat is mostly unsaturated. It's an inexpensive protein source with no cholesterol and could fit into a heart-healthy diet for adults. One tablespoon (fifteen ml) contains five grams of protein, some niacin, potassium, and magnesium, ninety-five calories and eight grams of fat. If the natural peanut butter is still too greasy for your taste, try spooning off some of the fat layer that rises to the top at room temperature. Add this lower-fat peanut butter to whole grain toast with jam for a combination that provides moisture with less fat.

Crackers Some crackers have as much fat as crisps. Read the label and watch for hydrogenated vegetable oil. If they leave a ring on your napkin or feel greasy to the touch, they will probably taste greasy and be high in fat. Gradually introduce some high-fibre crackers that are lower in fat. Concentrate on the crunch and taste of these crackers.

Cheese Check the label to find the amount of fat in the product. You will note that some of the higher-fat cheeses leave a sheen of grease on the surface when melted. As you begin to experiment with some of the lower-fat cheeses, you will note that they have a stringier texture and are great for holding the ingredients of a pizza in place.

Most cheeses labelled 'slender', 'lite', 'low-fat', or 'semi-skimmed' contain only slightly less fat than regular varieties. Even if a cheese has fifty percent less fat, as some labels promise, the fat is mostly saturated. This can account for sixty percent of the total calories. A popular cheese that claims to have twenty-five percent less fat than a regular brand contains 6.3 grams per serving rather than the 8.4 grams per serving in the regular version. This translates to sixty percent of the calories coming from fat rather than the sixty-eight percent in the regular brand. This is certainly not twenty-five percent less fat.

This doesn't mean that you should be eating only low-fat foods.

The idea is to increase your carbohydrate foods and gradually cut back on the fat used in food preparation. As your tastes begin to change, it will be more natural to choose prepared foods and meats with lower total fat content.

Remember, a healthy diet is all a matter of balance. Be careful not to totally avoid those foods that do not fit into the low-fat definition. If you approach label reading in this way you are right back into the diet thinking. Read the labels so that you will be aware of high-fat foods in order to continue guiding your preferences towards low-fat foods. As one of my clients put it, 'I didn't need self-control, I just needed to think normally. I have gained the ability to look at my eating as part of my life, not as an all-consuming hobby.'

SOME GUIDELINES TO HELP YOU ALONG IN YOUR PROCESS OF EXPERIMENTATION

- Cut down fat and sugar gradually so that you still enjoy eating the end product. For example, cutting the fat in half in your regular pie crust recipe and rolling the dough thinner with lattice crust on top (another option would be to use pastry cutters to cut out some of the top crust) results in a lighter pie crust that accents rather than detracts from the taste of the pie filling. Another tip would be to make the fruit filling thicker.

- To enhance the flavour, try other seasonings and flavourings. When cutting back on fat or sugar, adding more vanilla (i.e. doubling it) can bring out the flavour.

- To help moisten the recipe, try the addition of fruit or fruit juice. Fruit juice contains natural sugar, but the addition of liquid can also incorporate more moisture into the product.

- Sometimes words on labels may be misleading, for example, 'light'. There is no legislation to govern the use of this word. It may refer to the product being 'lighter' tasting, such as certain kinds of olive oil. It may refer to the product being 'lighter' in colour, such as certain kinds of soy sauce. Or it may refer to the product being lower in fat content such as certain kinds of mayonnaise.

'Light' yogurt, in spite of its name, is not low-calorie. It is a regular product at 260 calories per eight ounces (225 g) and it is sweetened with sugar. Ingredients read: low-fat milk, sugar, skimmed milk, strawberries, water, bananas, food starch (modified), yogurt culture, natural flavour, gelatin, citric acid, with sorbic acid and ascorbic acid (to ensure freshness), artificial colour.

Ensure that you always read the entire label carefully to determine its meaning. Today there is overuse of the words 'contains no cholesterol'. Here is an example.

The product may contain no cholesterol (for example, there may be no eggs in the product) but it may be high in saturated fat which has a greater effect on blood cholesterol levels as well as weight. As more consumers are catching on to the fact that the words 'no cholesterol' may be misleading, many manufacturers are attempting to lower the amount of saturated fat in the products. But we're still not getting the whole story. The product may in fact be low in cholesterol and saturated fat but high in total fat. Consumer beware!

Reading this front label leads you to believe that these biscuits are good for your heart and are healthy to eat. A closer look at the nutrition information per serving gives a very different picture. A serving of one biscuit contains thirty-four calories (these biscuits are very small). The biscuit has no cholesterol but it does contain two grams of fat. We know that there are nine calories per gram of fat so this equals 2×9 calories $= 18$ calories of the total thirty-four calories coming from fat (18 divided by $34 = 0.529 \times 100 = 53$ percent of calories in this biscuit come from fat). So these biscuits are high in fat which is going to affect both weight and cholesterol level.

Ingredients enriched wheat flour (wheat flour, niacin, reduced iron, thiamine mononitrate, riboflavin), sugar, vegetable shortening (partially hydrogenated soybean and/or cottonseed oil), rolled oats, chocolate chips, bran, raisins, corn syrup, honey, baking soda, salt, cinnamon, natural butter flavour, caramel colour.

THESE WORDS ALL MEAN 'SUGAR'

Brown sugar	A soft sugar whose crystals are covered by a film of refined dark syrup.
Carbohydrate	Sugars and starches.
Corn sugar	Sugar made by the breakdown of cornstarch.
Corn syrup	A syrup containing several different sugars that are obtained by the partial breakdown of cornstarch.
Dextrin	A sugar formed by the partial breakdown of starch.
Dextrose	Another name for sugar.
Fructose	The sweet sugar found in fruit, fruit juices, and honey.
Glucose	The type of simple sugar found in the blood, formed from food and used by the body for heat and energy.
Honey	A sweet thick material made in the honey sac of various bees; sweeter than sugar.
Invert sugar	A combination of sugars found in fruits.
Lactose	The sugar found in milk.
Levulose	Another name for fruit sugar.
Maltose	A crystalline sugar formed by the breakdown of starch.
Mannitol	A sugar alcohol.
Maple sugar	A syrup made by concentrating the sap of the sugar maple.
Molasses	The thick, dark to light brown syrup that is separated from raw sugar in sugar manufacture.
Sorbitol	A sugar alcohol.
Sorghum	Syrup from the juice of the sorghum grain (sorgo) grown mainly for its sweet juice.
Starch	A powdery complex sugar (carbohydrate), i.e. cornstarch.
Sucrose	Another name for sugar.
Sugar	A sweet carbohydrate.

Check the ingredients list. *Note* Even though the biscuits do not contain tropical oils (palm, coconut oils that are saturated), the third ingredient is vegetable shortening, a saturated fat that will affect blood cholesterol levels. The word hydrogenated in a product indicates hardened fat which makes the fat saturated. Even though the type of fat is from a vegetable source, it has been chemically altered through the process of adding hydrogen to the product which is called 'hydrogenation'. This process allows the product a longer shelf life and makes the fat hard at room temperature. Any positive effect of oat fibre on cholesterol levels is negated by the high amount of fat in the product.

Misleading labels and information can be confusing. In order to sell his product the food manufacturer has to make you want to buy it. Highlighting trendy information that will grab your attention is what he will aim to do.

Read the fine print as well and note where the different ways of saying 'fat' and 'sugar' appear on the label. However, ensure that you don't become preoccupied with the label. The product has to taste good and satisfy you.

ACTION POINTS

- Become more informed by reading food labels – in a non-obsessive way.

- Exercise your choice in purchasing products to suit your new tastes.

- Cut down on fats and sugars gradually.

- Experiment with seasonings and flavourings to enhance taste.

11

Fluids – How Much is Enough?

Are you really hungry or are you merely thirsty?

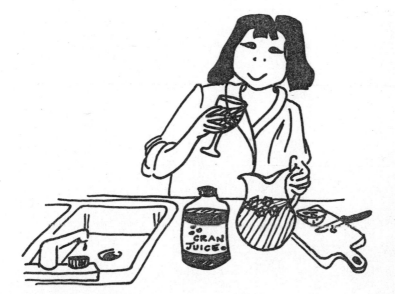

What kind of fluids could you be drinking and are they necessary for your health and wellbeing? Up to this point the discussion has centred on the techniques needed to tune in to our internal body signals to regulate hunger and the quantity of food your body needs. The act of tasting and savouring your food was also stressed because it allows you to be satisfied with less. Pausing during your meal allows you to stop and focus on your eating and consciously decide if you would like more, also allowing you to be satisfied with less.

Many people in the diet mentality fill up with water, coffee, or soup to lessen their hunger pangs temporarily. They are avoiding their natural hunger signals. Filling up with liquids instead of a meal makes them feel bloated and temporarily full. However, by the following meal, they may be famished and eat anything and everything.

Filling up on water prior to the meal is the diet method of dealing with hunger pangs. This makes you artificially full and you eat less at the meal. In other words, the bloating effect of the water causes you to eat less. This is not dealing with your physical hunger; it is avoiding the hunger or trying to dampen it artificially.

Our philosophy is to eat food when you are hungry and drink fluids when you are thirsty. If you try to trick your body by filling it up with fluids when you are actually hungry, it may work temporarily, but will lead to uncontrollable hunger later on.

Adequate fluid intake is important for your health and wellbeing. Using the technique of tuning in to your body to determine when you are thirsty is not as effective as it was for regulating hunger. Scientists don't yet fully understand how the thirst mechanism works. However, they do know that if you wait until you are thirsty, then you are partially dehydrated.

If you avoid your thirst signals you will eat more. All foods contain a certain amount of fluid. If you are not obtaining enough fluids from water or fruit juices to rehydrate your body's proper functioning, your body will signal you to eat more to obtain these fluids. If you go for a walk, and your natural cooling mechanism causes you to lose some water through perspiration, you need to rehydrate yourself when you come back.

Suppose you come back from your walk and see some watermelon in the fridge which contains ninety-two percent water. You are thirsty and it really looks good. You eat four slices to quench your thirst when really what your body wanted was water. Your fluids are replenished from food rather than from fluids. Unfortunately, you may end up even more thirsty due to the high-sugar content of the fruit.

The right strategy is to drink a sufficient amount of fluids, namely water, to rehydrate your body. If you still want the watermelon, have it after the fluid replacement, and you may actually be satisfied with less watermelon. Filling up on ice cream, popsicles, or a milkshake to cool you off and replace fluids does not address the real problem. These items are cold and they do not effectively replenish the fluids in your body. You may still be thirsty and feel unsatisfied.

SIGNS OF DEHYDRATION

How do you know if you are not consuming enough fluids? Watching for the signs of dehydration can give you the answer. Water is as critical to the body as oil is to a car's engine. The body needs fluids to function properly. Fluids allow reactions to take place in the body processes that keep you going.

Blood consists mostly of water and it carries oxygen and nutrients to your brain. Without enough water, you get a headache. This pain in your head is caused by insufficient oxygen, carried by water, to your brain. Dizziness and lack of concentration can also result if less nutrients and oxygen are carried to the brain.

Water is also the main ingredient in urine which carries wastes away from the body. Water is also needed to keep food moving through the intestinal tract and to help prevent constipation which may occur if you're eating high-fibre foods.

Without water we would die in a few days, yet we can live for weeks without food. A dark-coloured urine where only small amounts are eliminated is an indication of dehydration. If your body is not taking in sufficient fluids, it keeps you from becoming further dehydrated by releasing less water. Your urine is darker as it becomes more concentrated. Fluid retention may be another indication that your body is not taking in enough fluids. When the body gets less water, it perceives this as a threat to survival and begins to hold on to every drop. If you are taking vitamin pills, and you take in more than your body needs, the water-soluble vitamins B and C are passed through the urine, making it a darker colour. In this situation, colour would not be a good indicator of a state of hydration.

A weak fluttering pulse may be another sign of dehydration. A lower intake of water means that you will have less volume of blood. This will cause your heart to race or beat faster in order to pump the diminished supply of blood to your muscles.

Some water is produced as a by-product of metabolism. Six to eight glasses of liquid per day are usually needed to make up the balance. For example, under stressful situations, your blood becomes thicker once the reflex responses have kicked in. Drinking six to eight glasses of water per day can offer a protective effect since it dilutes your blood.

Water is particularly important for weight loss because it is necessary to help the body metabolise or break down fat. In short, water is necessary for your health and wellbeing. You know when you are dehydrated and consuming insufficient fluids; however, your thirst mechanism is not very sensitive in telling you when to drink fluids.

QUENCHING YOUR THIRST

Going from fizzy drinks or diet drinks to water is quite a drastic change. The more enticing fluids attract you because of their appeal to your senses of colour, flavour, and taste. You may shift to drinking water because you feel you should drink it, rather than because you enjoy water and like the taste of it. If you change to water gradually you will get used to it.

Let's take a look at the different types of liquids and their relationship to rehydrating you and quenching your thirst. Fluids listed as diuretic do not rehydrate you due to their effect of ridding the body of fluids by increasing urine production.

No more than two to three cups of coffee per day is recommended. Large amounts of coffee can cause diarrhoea while the tannins in tea may help stop simple diarrhoea.[1] Adding milk to the tea can bind the tannins and partly reduce their effect.

Drinking tea with meals can inhibit the absorption of iron from non-heme sources such as cereals and vegetables. One study showed that drinking tea with a meal decreases iron absorption by sixty-two percent.[2]

A mechanism by which tea is thought to influence iron absorption is by the formation of insoluble iron tannates. When milk is added to tea, the protein in milk reacts with the tannin in the tea and prevents the body from absorbing tannin. Adding milk to the tea binds the tannin, therefore improving the absorption of iron. Tannin in tea also slows the release of its caffeine and makes it a less immediate shock to the nervous system than the caffeine in coffee.

It was found that coffee may also decrease iron absorption, but not as much as tea. In a study done by Morck, Lynch, and Cook,[4] a cup of coffee (250 ml) reduced iron absorption from a hamburger meal by thirty-nine percent as compared to a sixty-four percent decrease with tea. This study suggests that reduced absorption was most marked when the coffee was taken with the meal or up to one hour later. A significant fraction of the meal would still be in the stomach after one hour and therefore the coffee would still decrease iron absorption.

Drinking coffee or tea before a meal or more than one hour after you finish eating will not interfere with iron absorption. Drinking fluids high in vitamin C such as juice spritzers (see p245) can enhance the absorption of iron from cereals and vegetables. (Refer to Chapter 4 for a list of foods high in vitamin C.)

Switching from coffee to tea provides a gradual drop in caffeine content. Since tea has about half as much caffeine as does coffee, withdrawal symptoms would be minimised. One way to test how addicted you are to caffeine is to try to stop using it for a day or two. Withdrawal symptoms are common. The first one to occur is usually a headache.

FLUIDS AND THEIR FUNCTIONS

Type of Beverage	Rehydration	Quenches Thirst
Coffee	No, it's a diuretic	Yes
Tea	No, it's a diuretic	Yes

Coffee and tea cause the blood vessels to dilate as the result of the xanthine content. Although caffeine is the strongest stimulant in coffee, tea, and cocoa, these drinks also contain other related xanthine compounds such as theophylline and theobromine that have similar, though less potent, effects. Caffeine is the main xanthine in coffee; but theophylline predominates in tea, and cocoa contains large amounts of theobromine. These chemicals contribute significantly to the stimulant effects of tea and cocoa.

Decaffeinated coffee	No, it's a diuretic	Yes

Note that decaffeinated coffee still contains two other stimulants called theophylline and theobromine. Cutting out coffee and tea can cause caffeine withdrawal symptoms such as headaches, so taper off coffee and tea consumption gradually. Switching from coffee to tea can lead to a gradual decrease in caffeine content. A 5-oz (150 ml) cup of strong tea brewed for five minutes contains 45 mg caffeine while a 5-oz (150 ml) cup of percolated coffee contains 110 mg caffeine. Use the substitution of tea for coffee only if you enjoy the taste of tea; otherwise, you may feel psychologically deprived by using what you would classify to be an inferior substitute.

Milk	No, net effect is dehydration due to high calcium and protein content	Yes
Soft drinks	Partially	No, due to high concentration of sugar, which makes you more thirsty.
Diet drinks	Yes	Somewhat

These drinks are artificially sweetened and have a sweet taste. Substituting these for regular drinks does not allow you to acquire a taste for less sugary foods. The increased consumption of artificially sweetened products has not decreased society's craving for sweets or the incidence of obesity. However, diet drinks do have their place. If you particularly like certain diet drinks, try adding a little water to them. Gradually increase the amount of water you add. This will allow you to achieve the goal of learning to acquire a taste for less sugary foods.

Fruit juices	Partially	No, high concentration of natural sugar, makes you more thirsty.

Drinking pop or fruit juices usually leaves you with the feeling of wanting more.

Alcohol	No	No

Even though alcoholic beverages are not diuretics, they do have a diuretic effect in that they increase urine production.[3] Alcohol inhibits the secretion of the antidiuretic hormone. During an alcoholic bout, lack of this hormone combined with the dilating of the vessels of the kidney add to this effect. The diuretic effect of alcoholic beverages can cause a state of dehydration commonly known as a hangover.

The headache typically begins with a sensation of fullness in the head and progresses to a painful throbbing that is made worse by bending over and by exercise. It is relieved by caffeine, or painkillers that contain caffeine such as Anacin or Excedrin. Caffeine is included in headache remedies to constrict blood vessels in the brain, since dilated blood vessels contribute to migraine-type headaches. Regular coffee drinkers who abstain from caffeine in the evening may wake up with a headache the next morning.

Other symptoms of caffeine withdrawal (or overdose) are:

- headache;

- drowsiness;

- lethargy;

- yawning;

- runny nose;

- irritability;

- disinterest in work;

- nervousness;

- mental depression;

- nausea; and

- vomiting.

Caffeine is one of the non-prescription mood-altering drugs. Abrupt withdrawal may mimic the symptoms of consuming too much caffeine.

In a study done at Johns Hopkins University, it was found that withdrawal symptoms began eighteen hours after caffeine intake, peaked at twenty-four hours, and then gradually decreased. Withdrawal symptoms included headache, fatigue, muscle stiffness and soreness (flu-like symptoms), and significant deterioration of mood and behaviour.

Further insight revealed that overnight abstinence from caffeine caused low-grade withdrawal symptoms. For this reason, taking coffee in the morning may give you a lift because it suppresses withdrawal symptoms. Caffeine drinkers are more lethargic and irritable in the morning before drinking coffee than are caffeine abstainers. Heavy consumption of caffeine is considered to be about eight cups (two L) of coffee per day. Moderate consumption is four cups (one L) of coffee or less per day.

Wean yourself off coffee gradually by decreasing the number of cups of coffee by one or two a day until you're down to a safe level of two to three cups (500 to 700 ml) a day. Switching to tea is a gradual reduction of caffeine. Eventually steep the bag for less time for less total caffeine content. Start switching to tea only if you enjoy the taste. Otherwise, you will be using it as a poor substitute for something you really like. The end result may be a feeling of deprivation, which is something you are striving to avoid. Another method would be to gradually mix more decaffeinated coffee into the pot brewed each morning.

Even though chocolate contains cocoa which contains caffeine, you would have to consume about half a pound (225 g) of dark chocolate and a pound or more (± 450 g) of milk chocolate to get the stimulant effect of one or two cups (250 to 500 ml) of brewed coffee.[5] Coffee is the main source of caffeine.

CAFFEINE CONTENT OF FOOD

SOURCE	AMOUNT	CAFFEINE
Brewed coffee	6 oz (175 ml)	66–180 mg
Instant coffee	6 oz (175 ml)	60–100 mg
Decaffeinated coffee	6 oz (175 ml)	2–5 mg
Tea (5-minute brew)	6 oz (175 ml)	79–110 mg
Tea (1-minute brew)	6 oz (175 ml)	20–45 mg
Colas	10 oz (300 ml)	22–50 mg
Chocolate milk	8 oz (250 ml)	2–7 mg
Hot chocolate drink	6 oz (175 ml)	6–30 mg
Milk chocolate	1 oz (28 g)	1–15 mg
Dark chocolate	6 oz (175 g)	5–35 mg
Baker's chocolate	1 oz (28 g)	26 mg

When you drink a cup of coffee, the caffeine enters your bloodstream, and you feel alert. When a healthy human adult consumes caffeine, about ninety-nine percent of it is absorbed, with peak blood levels reached within fifteen to forty-five minutes. Within three to seven-and-a-half hours you reach for another cup of coffee to get the same feeling back again. However, this effect can be achieved naturally through a healthy lifestyle. Because caffeine stimulates the body to release more glucose into the bloodstream, it can artificially give a mental lift to keep your energy level high. The sudden rise in your blood glucose causes your pancreas to oversecrete insulin which causes blood glucose levels to quickly drop. This is what makes you want another cup of coffee shortly after the first cup – to bring the blood glucose levels back up.

Are you 'jump starting' your body with caffeine instead of food? Needing that first cup of coffee to get you going signals a physical dependence on an unnatural stimulant. Natural stimulants such as physical activity and healthy eating decrease the dependence on these artificial stimulants.

Try eating a more substantial breakfast, followed by a single cup of coffee. This uses the beverage more for enjoyment than for a lift. Using coffee in the right way will allow you to enjoy it. Using it in place of food will not benefit your health. If you can't live without that cup of coffee first thing in the morning and use the stimulants in coffee to get you going, you are probably addicted.

TEA/HERBAL TEA

While many herbal teas are perfectly safe, others contain potent drugs that could prove more hazardous than caffeine. Herbal teas are popular because they are said to pick you up, calm you down, speed up or slow down the bowels, and even improve your sex life.

Treat herbs as drugs. They may have ingredients that affect the system in the same way that caffeine and alcohol do. These biologically active ingredients are usually present in low concentration so that drinking a little presents no noticeable problem. However, some teas are combinations of herbs that may increase or decrease the effect of a drug you are taking.

Some Rules of Thumb to Consider
- Read labels. If the herbal tea package doesn't list ingredients, don't buy it!

TEA INGREDIENTS CONSIDERED SAFE

Peppermint
Spearmint
Melissa or Balm
Dandelion
Red and Black Raspberry
Cayenne
Slippery Elm
Ginger
Rose hips (high in vitamin C) and hibiscus

None of these teas have been known to cause birth defects. Both rose hips and hibiscus have mild laxative and diuretic effects. There is no reason not to use them.

INGREDIENTS TO BE AVOIDED – DEADLY

St John's Wort
Golden Seal
Calamus Root
Sassafras or safrole

Sassafras tea is a mild stimulant that contains a potent cancer-causing compound known as safrole. Prior to 1960, it had been widely available. It is available today in health food stores.

SEVERE DIURETICS OR STRONG LAXATIVES

Juniper Berries
Shave Grass (Horsetail)
Buckthorn Bark
Senna Leaves, Flowers
Dock (Burdock)
Aloe Leaves and Bark
Alfalfa Tea (in excess)

MIND-ALTERING

Hyssop
Juniper
Catnip
Hydrangea
Kavabava
Lobelia
Jimsonweed
Wormwood
Nutmeg in high doses

These teas affect the central nervous system. Typical symptoms are blurred vision, dry mouth, inability to urinate, bizarre speech and behaviour, including hallucinations.

ALLERGIC REACTIONS

Yarrow
German and
Roman Camomile
Goldenrod
Marigold

These teas should be avoided by sensitive persons such as those allergic to ragweed. For all persons they should be consumed in moderation only, not more than two cups (500 ml) per day and not on a daily basis.

OTHER TEAS TO AVOID

Ginseng*
Fennel*
Liquorice Root***

*These have hormone-like effects such as painful or swollen breasts even in men. Prolonged use (over six months) may cause insomnia, diarrhoea, and depression.
***In large amounts, tea may cause water and sodium retention, possible high blood pressure, and even cardiac arrest.

- Not all herbal teas are caffeine-free. Herb or spice blends that contain black tea or green tea have caffeine.

- Introduce a new tea slowly. Brew weak tea at first. Allow the tea to steep for a few minutes then remove the herbs. Drink only in moderation until the tea's effect on you is known to be safe.

- Brew fresh tea each time, since active chemicals are slowly leached from the plant as it steeps.

- Listen to your body. Try half a cup (125 ml) of weak tea the first time, and if it has no ill effect, you might try a full cup the next time.

Putting the Zip in Tea: a Safer Alternative

Tea is a sensible alternative to soft drinks and coffee. After water, it is the most reasonably priced beverage, costing just a few pence a cup. *Note* For weaker tea with less caffeine, brew for less time. Adding fruit juice to the tea adds some flavour, dilutes the caffeine in the tea and decreases the diuretic effect of the tea.

Adding more variety and interest to your beverages allows you to get more psychological benefits from fluids. Here are some ideas to use tea as a more exotic beverage.

- Combine equal amounts of freshly brewed tea and warm apple juice. Sprinkle with cinnamon and nutmeg or include a cinnamon stick. This is especially good for those trips in winter when you take along a hot thermos of your favourite drink. The flavour from the cinnamon stick will leach into the water.

- Hot tea plus a few teaspoons (ml) each of lemon and honey is a favoured remedy for sore throats any time of year. To make it extra special, top it off with a twist of lemon peel.

- Freshly brewed cup of tea plus 1 tsp (5 ml) grated orange peel and a cinnamon stick to garnish.

- Freshly brewed cup of tea plus 1/4 tsp (1 ml) each of vanilla and almond extract.

- Freshly brewed tea plus fruit juices. Try pineapple, grapefruit, or orange juice, half and half, with hot tea. Garnish with lemon or orange slice.

- For a hot vegetable sipper, combine 1/2 cup (125 ml) freshly brewed tea with 1/2 cup (125 ml) warm vegetable cocktail juice. Season with 1 tsp (5 ml) Worcester sauce.

- Equal portions of hot tea plus warm pineapple juice plus a few lightly crushed cardamom pods. The aroma is wonderful; the taste is sensational.

- Weak tea with a twist of lemon. Served with plenty of ice.

The fruit juices provide some of the natural sweetness. Add sugar or honey to sweeten, if desired. Keep in mind that you gradually want to acquire a taste for less sugary foods. The fruit juice provide sweet calories from the natural sugar, so check carefully. Do you really want that extra sugar or is it purely habit?

CAFFEINE AND WEIGHT

Can drinking more coffee burn fat? Here's the answer you've been waiting for. Caffeine raises the metabolic rate which means that you will burn more calories at rest. Caffeine is also known to burn more fat during exercise. It does this by sparing glycogen, your carbohydrate stores, and using fat as a fuel source. The down side of caffeine consumption is that it triggers the release of insulin which causes blood sugar to drop, as discussed earlier in this chapter.

As you know, when your blood sugar is low, you are hungry. You eat more, replacing the fat that you lost. Increasing your caffeine content does not give you any overall weight loss benefit. As for increased endurance that occurs by sparing glycogen and using fat as a fuel source, this will be offset if too much caffeine is consumed. It is known that athletes who drink three to four large mugs of coffee before competition become so hyper they perform poorly.

Normally when on a diet, a person switches from regular drinks to diet drinks. But is this learning to acquire a taste for less sugary foods? You still crave sweet foods even though you substitute a diet item for the regular one. Studies have shown that switching to diet products is not decreasing the evidence of obesity.

Our society used to be concerned with sugar. Now sugar is no longer so bad; it is fat that is the culprit. Yet there is no such thing as a perfect way of eating and no food is good or bad. It is the food balance that is important so that you minimise the starve/binge cycle.

Diet thinking suggests that you are allowed to eat more if the product contains fewer calories. 'I'll eat a big supper and finish off with an artificial sweetener in my coffee.' This all-or-nothing thinking is predominant in our society.

Carol used to drink diet drinks all the time and she relied on diet products. She couldn't understand why she always craved sweets when she saw them and she binged on them at social occasions. Possibly it was because the artificially sweetened foods still allowed her to like the sweet taste. However, by gradually adding water to her beverages, Carol learned to acquire a taste for less sugary foods. She still likes chocolate cake but now a few bites will satisfy her. She actually finds the cake too sweet. The goal is to change your taste rather than simply reduce the calorie intake which does not address the real problem.

When blood sugar is low, you are hungry, tired, lack energy, and feel irritable. This lowers your level of productivity, decreasing your ability to concentrate. You may turn to foods or beverages that lessen these symptoms temporarily (coffee and doughnuts) but end up sending your blood sugar on a roller coaster ride. This scenario is part of the 'office syndrome'. It is typical of many people in our society.

John stayed up late last night, eating crisps while watching the late film on TV. He felt rushed this morning and had no time for breakfast. He didn't feel hungry anyway. He grabbed a cup of coffee and a doughnut at work. Then he felt better and ready for a day's work. By ten o'clock he was feeling tired and hungry. John thought he shouldn't eat any more so he had another cup of coffee. That kept him going until lunchtime.

However, at lunchtime he felt starved and had a headache. He gulped his food so fast that there was little consciousness of what he ate and he neither tasted nor savoured the food. He had room for dessert so ate it, rationalising that he hadn't eaten much earlier on so he deserved it. He ended the meal with two cups of coffee to get him going for the afternoon. By mid-afternoon he felt sluggish. Since he overate at lunch he felt he shouldn't eat any more. He compensated for overeating by having only a cup of coffee to give him a boost. The coffee gave him an immediate surge of energy but then he felt wiped out. His head was pounding.

By supper time, John was too tired to prepare a decent supper. He ate some biscuits and plonked himself in front of the TV. He was tired of fighting the overpowering cravings and dealing with his wildly erratic energy levels.

Why was this happening to John? Poor eating habits caused him to depend on caffeine rather than food for energy. The choice of doughnuts provided an immediate burst of energy from the carbohydrates but fifty percent of these calories came from fat. Combined with caffeine which also resulted in a sudden increase in blood sugar, the foods gave a surge of insulin, resulting in a sudden drop in blood sugar.

ENJOYING THE TASTE OF WATER

People do not drink simply to quench their thirst; they respond to a need that's as much in the mind as in the body. Psychological satisfaction is the reason they drink (often something other than water) even if they're not really thirsty. They may simply want to enjoy the taste of the beverage. Presentation of drinks and flavour combinations that excite the eye as well as the palate go a long way towards giving a person psychological satisfaction from drinks. Serving drinks in tall, fancy glasses or using a carafe full of a colourful drink with ice is appealing to the eye. Try making your drink special. You are worth it.

Just as you gradually decrease the fat content of foods you choose, you can gradually add water to beverages to learn to acquire a taste for less sugary drinks. Diet drinks do not help you to resist the inevitable binge on sweets at a social function if you have not conquered your craving for sweets.

Non-dieters are more selective and eat only what they really like. If you learn to acquire a taste for less sugary foods, then you may choose to omit some or have only a few bites since the food will taste too sweet to you. The end result is that you eat less because you choose to eat less, not because you feel you should stop eating sweets but because you do not crave them. You will eat only what you really want.

Eating more carbohydrates that break down into natural sugar will allow you to crave fewer sweets. Restricting carbohydrates causes your body's natural defence mechanism to kick in to make you crave the sweets so that you obtain the energy source from these foods.

Gradually add water to any fruit juices, drinks, or diet drinks that you are now using as part of your fluid intake. This can also apply to coffee or tea. Eventually you will end up with coloured water that will taste refreshing and will rehydrate you more effectively as well as quench your thirst.

Mary didn't like orange juice because she found it too acidic. By adding more water than the directions specified, she made a taller drink, cut the acidity, got vitamin C, and at the same time quenched her thirst. She also began to enjoy foods that did not taste as sweet.

FLAVOURED SELTZERS, FRUIT SPRITZERS, OR REFRESHERS

*These creations quench thirst and also appeal to
the eye and taste buds.*

Start with 2/3 cup (150 ml) beverage or juice and 1/3 cup (75 ml) water, then go to 1/2 cup (125 ml) beverage or juice and 1/2 cup (125 ml) water a week or two later, followed by 1/4 cup (50 ml) juice or beverage and 3/4 cup (175 ml) water a few weeks later, until you reach the level that works for your taste buds and psychological satisfaction. By doing this you don't add substantial 'sugar' calories to your waist, and you quench your thirst as well.

FRUIT SPRITZERS & REFRESHERS

- Combine different fruit juices and add ice cubes and spring water. Add slices of lemon or lime or a squirt of lemon or lime concentrate. Diluting lime cordial is another option.

- Spring water with ice and a squirt of lemon or lime is refreshing.

- Start with different cranberry versions of cocktail juices. Cranberry and apple, cranberry and raspberry, and cranberry and grape add colour and flavour to your drinks. Gradually add more water. Blackcurrant or raspberry cocktail can also make a refreshing drink.

- Invent your own flavoured drinks. For example, mix a few drops of grenadine or blackcurrant syrup with water, and serve with fruit slices.

- Fruit juice spritzers are delicious. Try grape spritzer. Use 1/4 cup (50 ml) unsweetened white grape juice; 3/4 (175 ml) cup bottled spring water alone or with some diet 7up. The bottled water will dilute the sweet taste of the diet 7up so you are still learning to acquire a taste for less sugary foods by using the diet drinks in this way.

- Lemonade spritzer can be made from bottled water or ice and regular water added to lemonade. Water will cut the strong concentrated flavour of the lemon but leave the 'punch' and appeal.

- Wine spritzers or light beers or diluted liqueurs are enjoyable.

- Try a shandy. Mix half beer and half ginger ale or lemonade. Add a little lime juice or lemon juice if you like. Try your shandy with light beer.

- Sangria is made from red or white wine with ice. Add spring water and fruit such as strawberries, lemon, lime, or orange pieces, some root beer, coke, or lemonade.

- Effervescent drinks (soda or diet drinks) can add bubbles to your juice spritzers instead of using bottled water and save you money at the same time.

- Squeeze an orange or lemon into iced water and add some slices or slivers of orange or lemon for a fast drink.

- Add celery sticks to water. The flavour will leach into the water with time, leaving a refreshing taste.

WINTER SEASON DRINK SUGGESTION

- Add water to apple juice with a cinnamon stick or a dash of cinnamon. Heat it up in the microwave.

- Any of the refreshers on p245 can be heated up for a warmer drink for the winter.

- Try various fruit combinations of tea. The less time you allow the tea to steep in the water, the lower the caffeine content. Add fruit spritzer to regular tea for another version of a hot drink.

- Hot milk with a dash of instant coffee or a squirt of liqueur can be used for a special occasion. If you would like the alcoholic content to go, add liqueur to milk, and then heat it up. In this way, you get the benefit of the flavour without the alcohol.

Another idea is to try beverages, including water, at different temperatures. For some people, having a beverage too cold or too hot may not allow them to extract the true taste and enjoyment from the liquid. This is true even with water.

Water doesn't have to be boring. By creating some excitement with beverages, you will drink more fluids and eat because of physical hunger, rather than because your body needs to replenish the fluids. Use your imagination with drinks. Fine-tune your fluid concoctions just as you did your present recipes.

Drinking plenty of water to rehydrate your body after exercising is important; otherwise you may feel dizzy because your body is pumping a diminished supply of blood to the brain. Use the technique of confrontation to determine whether you are really hungry or simply thirsty. Tuning into your signals for thirst may not be as effective as tuning into your hunger signals. When you drink, your thirst will feel quenched long before your fluid loss is replenished. This is especially pronounced during physical activity when you may become significantly dehydrated before you feel thirsty. It's possible to lose up to two quarts (2.3 L) of water before you notice your fluid loss. This is why it is important to drink water before, during, and after exercise in cold weather and in hot. Increase your fluid intake between meals and determine whether it helps you to actually eat less.

Dieters tend to drink fluids prior to meals hoping this will cause them to fill up on liquids. This in turn may make them eat less simply because they are temporarily more bloated. It leads to increased hunger later on once this feeling subsides.

When increasing the fibre content of your meals, water is essential because high-fibre foods absorb water. In order for foods such as whole grains to allow you to relieve constipation, enough water must be consumed. Increased intake of water in itself will help to improve your bowel movements.

ACTION POINTS

● Ensure fluid intake is adequate – six to eight glasses a day is usually needed.

● Tune in to the different feelings of hunger and thirst.

● Watch out for signs of dehydration.

● Pay particular attention to fluid requirements when exercising.

● Gradually cut down on tea and coffee consumption.

● Develop a taste for water.

● Experiment with different 'cocktails' of water and fruit juices to make drinks more appealing.

● Notice the difference between the drinks that actually quench your thirst and those that hydrate you.

12

Lifestyle Strategies

Take time for yourself and relax.

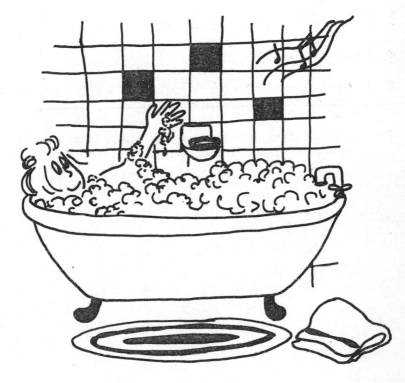

BUILDING RELAXATION INTO YOUR LIFE

'I do not have any time for myself. I have a career, family commitments, and a partner. Taking care of their needs absorbs all my time. It leaves nothing for me.' This situation is common with today's working mothers. Although many women work outside the home, to a great degree the responsibility of family and household care may still be theirs. The result is burnout, a deprivation of time for themselves. They become both physically and emotionally drained and have no way to renew their energies.

Special time for yourself should focus on an activity that you enjoy. What do you really want to do?

- go for a walk, some quiet time to close your eyes and daydream or take yourself away to a place you would like to be (visualisation);

- read a book or newspaper;

- have a snack to take care of your hunger when you come home from work;

- have a bubble bath;

- do a crossword puzzle;

- listen to classical music; or

- do stretching exercises, and/or deep breathing.

How can you create time for yourself? There are demands on your time as soon as you walk in the door. Plan carefully to reserve some time to attend to your own needs.

Lisa said, 'Everybody is hungry when I come home and they want to eat right away so they can get on with their activities.' You are worn out trying to attend to everyone. And if you are constantly running on low energy, tired, and irritable, your quality of life and that of your family suffers. One solution would be to make it known that you need a half hour to yourself when you get home from work. Or perhaps you are a victim of the arsenic hour, that hour before supper when the kids are dogging your footsteps, they're cranky, and they don't stop pestering you. Perhaps they are simply experiencing low blood sugar. They are probably hungry. Putting the meal in front of them immediately seems the easiest solution, but to do that you must forfeit the special time you need for your own wellbeing. Does it sound like a dilemma?

Perhaps there is a solution. A handy snack to dampen immediate hunger pangs will allow the children to be in a state of 'pleasant hunger' so they are more likely to taste and savour their meal. The added bonus is that they will be in a better frame of mind to enjoy supper. This will also eliminate that 'Mum, I'm hungry,' an hour after supper is over.

The snack could consist of celery sticks with quark cheese, fruit, milk, crackers and cheese, toast with peanut butter and jam, or any other of their favourite foods. Snacks can even be prepared after supper for the next day while you are still working in the kitchen. To make this process even simpler, have easy ready-made purchased snacks handy. Try seasoned bread sticks, melba toast, cheese and crackers, yogurt, milk, bread, rolls, or fruit.

As the children get older, they can take responsibility for the snacks themselves. The years when you prepared the snacks could serve as an example for them to follow. This creates independence and frees more time for Mum.

While you are resting let the oldest child be in charge for the first half hour and make the others aware that they are to sit quietly and colour or watch television. Once a routine is established they will accept it.

Your special time is for you and you alone. In order to avoid noise and distraction you may want to go for a walk to collect your thoughts, regain your composure, and put the sanity back into your life. The real benefit of building a daily relaxation period into your life is that you are not exhausted by the time your holiday time comes around. Holidays become a pleasure instead of a necessity to relieve your exhaustion.

People often go to extremes. They work too hard and play too hard as well. If they dine out they overeat, and tend to eat and drink too much at parties. The balance is gone from life.

By building in a daily 'time off' period, you can regain the relaxed composure necessary to enjoy the moment so that you can eat your meal or listen to your children. You can give them your interested attention. You become more focused and a better listener. You also become more efficient because you focus on the situation and enjoy it.

If you don't take the time out to renew your energy you sap your reserves by continuing to overwork your body and mind. You feel overwhelmed most of the time and this causes further energy drain. It's time to take charge and do something positive rather than continue to complain about your situation. Don't wait until you are burned out and your body forces you to stop working. Listen to your body so that you can pull back, recharge, and maintain the balance between health and vigour.

Society's demands, pressures of the job, your own high expectations create a high stress level for you. Your own attitude towards a situation, the necessity of doing everything right the first time, and unrealistic goals and aspirations can aggravate the stress level.

Of course, you want to strive to be the best that you can be. Your inner strength comes from acknowledgement of your own self-worth. So be nice to yourself. Don't use failures to whip yourself. Use them instead as stepping stones to something better. You can do this if you retain a balance in life. So do not compromise your relaxation time. If you do, it will drain your energy reserves and cause you to be less efficient and productive.

Taking time out allows you to focus more on the event as you are doing it. Do you find you are absent-minded? If you are concentrating on supper when you put your wallet down, you may spend a lot of time looking for it the next time you want it. Why? Because you were living for the future, instead of the present. You were not thinking of where you were putting your wallet when you put it down and so when it comes time to find it, you don't know where it is.

You, not outside events, control how extensively stress affects your life. Stress is your response to the situation, not the situation itself. For example, if you get stuck in traffic, an event that is out of your control, you can choose to get annoyed and yell at anyone who beeps his horn. Or you can view the time you're sitting there as the only uninterrupted fifteen minutes you'll have all day, a time to reflect, a time to turn on some classical music. It's all a matter of attitude and how you handle the situation.

Building in time for yourself helps to stop that rushed feeling and allows you to do things more systematically, thinking of what you are doing while you are doing it. It puts you in a more relaxed frame of mind for mealtime. You can enjoy the meal rather than feel 'Let's get it over with so that I can finally relax.'

The rushed way of thinking involves doing things to extremes, getting everything done, so you can relax. This approach is unhealthy, unbalanced, and self-defeating. When you rush in order to relax, you then find you're too tired or too edgy to relax. You are living for the future when you will have 'time off' rather than enjoying each moment and living it comfortably at a level that you are able to handle. Living in any other time than the present produces stress. Work on finding ways to let this renewed energy and feeling of being in charge work for you daily, not only when you're on holiday.

Waiting until holiday time to relax can leave you burned out during the year. To prevent this, build in daily mini-relaxation breaks and short weekend getaways for that circuit-breaker when you simply need a little re-energising. Then your longer holidays will be a pleasure not a necessity. They will get you away from work and home and allow you to relax completely. All of these rechargers can restore the balance in your life.

Allow spontaneity and adventure a place in your life. A last-minute spontaneous weekend getaway that allows you to explore new territory, get some fresh air, and be active can sometimes be an effective pick-up and do you as much good as a month-long holiday. Make the most of what is available to you!

Observe those around you who have the ability to relax naturally. Peter relaxes by going downstairs and listening to classical music. After a while he feels regenerated. Interestingly enough, even though he frequently consumes high-fat foods, his cholesterol level is normal. He knows how to 'let go' of daily problems. He puts them on hold and his attitude towards life is upbeat and positive.

His wife, Louise, also leads a healthy lifestyle, eats in a healthy manner, and has become a non-smoker. However, her preoccupation with eating perfectly and making the right choices along with a difficulty in scheduling time out for herself may result in a higher risk of heart disease. Acquiring a taste for new interests such as learning how to listen to music and appreciate it could help her relax. Or she could build in some other form of activity that she enjoys to regenerate herself and give her more energy.

If you find it difficult to relax, take time to eat, breathe deeply, or have a nap and you find these activities unproductive and a waste of time, try to make yourself do them. Introduce them gradually. Taking the time to relax can serve to recharge your battery. People who exhibit the 'hurry-up' behaviour, called Type A personality, are seven to ten times more likely to develop heart disease than are their more relaxed counterparts.

At a presentation I heard about a study done in England where 200 participants were divided into two groups. One hundred participants were the control group and the other hundred were asked to have a half-hour nap sometime during the day. The latter group decreased their risk of heart disease by thirty percent. A little pause during the day can go a long way for health. Next time you feel you'd like to lie down for a nap, don't feel guilty. It may help you to regenerate yourself.

Tim works hard and enjoys his hobby. Taking time out for crossword puzzles and jigsaw puzzles allows him to acquire new concentration skills and extended vocabulary while relieving some of the pressure of everyday life. The relaxed disposition of people like Tim is apparent in their ability to handle stressful situations. So, as you've observed and learned from non-dieters, try to observe those who have the ability to relax naturally and learn how they do it. These people seem to be able to react positively even in negative situations. You can benefit from them.

You can make eating a positive experience. By learning to focus on eating, you will be celebrating food, and you will derive both psychological and physical satisfaction from the activity. If you've been eating in a rushed manner for years, you might ask, 'How do I go about tasting my food? How can I take time to spend time eating?'

Wait a minute. Are you feeling that you are not worth the time? Do you ever consider that by focusing on what you are doing while you are doing it you will actually free more quality time for you and your family? Taking time to enjoy your meal and making it a pleasurable dining experience can make your meals 'special'.

Tasting and savouring your food allows you to focus on your eating while you are eating and therefore you feel as if you have actually eaten a meal when you have finished. When you do this it disrupts the automatic eating that leads to taking in more than your body needs or wants. It also prevents constant nibbling throughout the day and evening. You will have more time as your new focus on food will transfer to other activities so that you begin to do all things more systematically. For example, concentrating on where you put your keys when you put them down will allow you to find them again when you want them without wasting time.

These preparations and skills will help you focus on eating while you are eating.

- Adopt a new attitude towards eating. Attitude can be defined as the way you think, feel, and act. For example, if you are dreading eating, or simply eating to consume food and get it over with, you are not deriving physical or psychological benefit from food. You may be focusing on what you will be doing after eating, rather than celebrating the act of eating itself. Enjoy the act of eating your food.

- Create a more relaxed atmosphere in which to eat your food. Do this by breaking the constant rush of the day's activities. If you are pressured all day and come home only to hurry to feed yourself and your family, the enjoyment of the meal is gone. Everybody feels tense. Relax when you come home before having your meal, then actually enjoy the meal together as a family.

- Many things can help you celebrate food. Present the food in an attractive way. Colour, texture, and aroma can highlight the experience of eating. Make every meal an event to enjoy, an occasion to anticipate. Special dishes, tablecloths, candles help to create a special atmosphere and need not be restricted only to holidays. Create more special days throughout the year by adding these trimmings.

With more rest time, you will be happier and more energetic. By building in that time-off for yourself, you are allowing yourself to be 'special'. You will no longer feel controlled by the whims of others. As you relax, you will give people more of your time because you want to, not simply because of duty or necessity.

The bonus for you is that you break the rushing syndrome and create a more relaxed atmosphere to enjoy eating at mealtime. Allowing yourself to have a snack between lunch and supper if you are actually hungry prevents you from coming to the table famished and eating out of control.

COMPARING DIETER'S AND NON-DIETER'S APPROACH TO MEALS

The Dieter's Approach
Not hungry in the morning. Got to run so you dash out the door with no breakfast. Your system is used to it. The day is busy, packed full of work and decisions to be made. Can't stop for lunch; otherwise you won't be able to complete the work. You work through lunch. You will be having a big supper so you'd better not overdo it by eating a big lunch. You grab a chocolate bar on the way home for quick energy in order to cope with the excitement at home. You feel edgy and when your kids are hungry, tired, and irritable and make demands on you, you feel drained. Somehow you manage to find the energy to make supper. It's one more job to be done before you can actually relax. You live for seven o'clock. You rush through supper so that you can get the dishes done and finally relax. You plonk on the sofa at seven-thirty. You turn on the television, feel hungry again since you ate so quickly, and go to the kitchen to fix yourself a snack. Peace at last.

Analysing the Situation

Nibbling in the evening can dampen your hunger for breakfast. You could try to eat in such a way that you are hungry at breakfast time. That may mean trying to forgo your evening snack or to make it smaller. Eating breakfast essentially 'breaks' the 'fast' and gets your system revved up to begin the day.

Since you seem to focus on total time rather than efficient time, you have skipped lunch because you were busy. Thinking more clearly about making your time more valuable and more productive through healthy eating and activity can improve your focus and productivity. It is not the total amount of time that counts, but what you accomplish with the time available.

Nibbling or not eating through the day to compensate for a larger meal in the evening causes your battery to run low all day. That is the diet mentality. The chocolate bar that you eat for a pick-up gives you a caffeine and sugar boost. The effects are almost immediate because you consume it on an empty stomach. However, the boost doesn't last long. The caffeine in the cocoa and sugar in the bar result in an immediate quick increase in blood sugar that sends your blood sugar tumbling again due to oversecretion of insulin by the pancreas.

The result is that you are 'wiped out' (fatigue, irritability) as you wait for the day to end. You are definitely not equipped to handle the situation at home. You have low energy, little tolerance and extreme hunger. You may grab anything in sight or end up nibbling as you prepare supper. If you are focusing on the needs of your family, you deprive yourself of the proper nourishment of mind and body that could restore your balance. You may actually resent the fact that you have to spend the time to prepare a meal and you may resort to convenience foods. High fat and little taste and flavour may cause you to feel that you missed out on the enjoyment of the meal that you were looking forward to all day. Then you eat sweets to compensate for your disappointment.

The entire day has been out of balance and this leads to the final let-down at the end of the day. You may continue in this manner day after day and miss out on the pleasure of living.

A healthier version of the same scenario puts you in control of your life by putting the balance back into it.

The Non-dieter's Approach

Using a non-dieter's approach, this scenario could occur more frequently.

You know that tomorrow will be an extremely busy day. Getting up a few minutes earlier seems impossible so you pack yourself some breakfast the night before. Depending on the time, you may decide to eat it before you leave for work, in the cafeteria at work if you arrive a little early, or at your first coffee break. Even though your day is busy, you make sure you take time for lunch. The pause in your busy schedule plus the lunch helped you to refocus for the decision-making in the afternoon. Because you felt regenerated you accomplished more productive work during the rest of the day.

Feeling hungry on the way home, you ate some crackers stored in the glove compartment of your car. This helped dampen the feelings of hunger that you usually experience at this time. When you arrive home, your kids have eaten the snacks you left for them. You have established a half hour for yourself and the kids do not bother you. You relax and leave behind the rushed feelings you had at work. You are entitled to this.

You remember that your father took time before supper to read the paper or lie down and your mother made sure you that did not bother him for at least half an hour to an hour after he came home from work. The difference then was that your mother was working in the home and helped build this balance into your home life. Now with women working outside the home, they also need this transitional time to unwind; otherwise they will become burned out.

Depending on how you feel, you may choose to have another small snack, go for a walk and reflect on the day's activities, read a magazine, or lie down. You close the book on your work activities and plan for family activities. You may decide to put supper in the oven while you relax in your free time. If the children are old enough they can be responsible for supper or your partner can take a turn.

Rather than dreading supper, with this scenario you look forward to it and enjoy the occasion. You value this family time and treasure mealtimes to review family activities. The above scenario allows you to put the balance back in your life, and to be happier and more productive.

Let's review the steps you took.

- You had a snack to dampen your hunger before supper (that is, if you were hungry between meals).

- You built in some time for yourself to create the proper atmosphere for eating.

- You are learning to focus on your eating while you are eating.

Aim to put relaxation into your lifestyle. A rushed lifestyle leads to rushed eating. Taking a few moments to relax prior to eating can put you in a more relaxed frame of mind to enjoy your meal. If you don't take the time to enjoy and savour your food, it can cause automatic 'nibbling' later on because you will still be looking for satisfaction from food.

- Use the breathing technique explained later in this chapter if you feel anxious or as a way of building in the pause to relax.

- Sit down for a few minutes prior to preparing supper to read the paper, daydream, have a snack, go over the day's activities, go for a short walk (while supper is cooking).

- Leaving relaxation time only until the end of the day is the all-or-nothing thinking of dieters comparable to having a reward, probably food, at the end of the day. Building in relaxation more regularly in the form of short breaks, for example, will allow you to focus on your work and be more productive.

Pamper yourself. You're worth it and you'll feel better for it.

EATING AND ITS ASSOCIATIONS

Jean had a good business meeting and accomplished many things. She felt wonderful and on her way home stopped at the convenience store to pick up a bag of crisps. As she turned off the ignition, she realised that she usually rewarded herself with food whenever she felt she had accomplished something. She confronted the situation and realised that the accomplishment itself was the reward. It was an internal reward.

Many people reward themselves with food when they feel either happy or sad and rob themselves of the experience of the emotion itself. It's normal to feel depressed when something goes wrong. Many people try to see the positive in the situation by allowing themselves to feel the emotion and work it through. Talking to others about it helps you to see the situation in a more objective framework.

Building in relaxation time for yourself can help you to focus on becoming more aware of activities that may be associated with eating. A quick form of relaxation is deep breathing. It is a skill that, if practised when you are not stressed, can do wonders for you in stressful situations. Take a few minutes daily to practise it. It will help you to build the pause into situations naturally as you master the skill.

MAKING THE MOST OF DEEP BREATHING

The following technique is a skill that will help you to relax. It is very effective if you practise it regularly so that you are prepared to use the skill when you are under stress. It can help you when you feel anxious which may cause you to want something sweet to eat or smoke a cigarette to calm you.

Deep breathing is also a way of taking time for yourself. Don't feel guilty when you take time to practise this technique. The little time you are taking will help you to put the 'pause' into your lifestyle and help you to refocus and re-energise.

In order to get the most out of the technique, it is essential to understand the purpose of the inhalation and exhalation phase.

The inhalation phase is invigorating, tension-producing and is used somewhat like a yawn. When you are ready to finish an exercise, a deep breath or two will create tension and help bring you back to your normal level of alertness. It is used to come out of the relaxed state, and is usually combined with the flexing and stretching of muscles (i.e. as if you are awakening from a state of sleep).

The exhalation phase is relaxing and promotes a feeling of

sinking down, slowing down, and heaviness leading to a feeling of complete relaxation.

Technique

- Inhale slowly and steadily through the nose, expanding your abdominal area rather than the rib cage. (Many people do this incorrectly by sucking in their stomachs when they breathe in.) When you permit your body to inhale by itself without any conscious thought on your part, you will do it naturally and correctly.

- Focus your attention on the exhalation phase of the breathing cycle. Concentrate on it and think about it, exhaling slowly, and allowing the abdominal area to contract naturally. It is during this phase that you feel and experience the sensations described under 'exhalation phase' that will result in an overall state of relaxation.

- The key to this exercise is to feel the sensations as you exhale, and only on the exhalations.

Practising this technique will enable you to relax quickly at a moment's notice.

FOOD ASSOCIATIONS

Sometimes associations can trigger a desire to eat. You may not actually be hungry but feel compelled to eat anyway. You may be eating and not be conscious that you are doing it. For example, you may be watching television and eating peanuts or crisps compulsively, not even remembering tasting them. This is a form of automatic eating.

If you are not tasting the food, then it becomes wasted calories that will only end up on your waist. This form of eating is more a habit than a need or desire. You somehow associate television with eating. However, some of these associations may be so ingrained that you do not recognise what is happening. Ten pounds later your trousers no longer fit.

Earlier I spoke about eating as a temporary relief from stress, and I tried to deal with the reasons behind the eating, using positive techniques to overcome the negative situation.

Some activities associated with eating are also automatic. These are triggers that lead to eating where the focus is on the activities rather than on the food. Here is a list of possible activities.

- watching television;

- reading a book, magazine, or newspaper;

- social occasions where everyone else is eating;

- associating certain individuals with certain foods; and

- using food as a comforter to restore warm feelings when you are feeling low.

As society moves from the industrial age to the information age, keeping abreast of news and recent happenings in your field becomes a greater priority. Reading the newspaper or watching television while eating may be timesaving to accomplish two things at once. Are you really enjoying either event to its fullest?

The other scenario may be that you are exhausted after work and have only enough energy to watch television. You sit in front of television in the evenings hoping to unwind. You may come home from work too tired to make supper and you use convenience foods to prepare a quick meal. However, your poor eating habits give you less energy. The high-fat content of convenience foods may weigh you down and make you more sluggish. Plus there is very little psychological satisfaction from this food. You feel too tired to move, so there is no energy or time to do any physical activity.

Time, or lack of it, seems to be used as an excuse for being sedentary. You may not even perceive activity to be important enough to make an effort. Yet the extra energy that you can retrieve from regular activity can give you more time by improving your efficiency during the day and evening. It is not the number of hours worked but the amount accomplished that counts. You can look busy without accomplishing very much. Productivity is what really matters.

What is the common factor in these two situations? In both

instances, attention is on the television set, not the food. Over time these television/food associations become so strong that they may seem impossible to break. However, your new way of thinking will find these sedentary activities less enjoyable.

Bob's situation is an example. Bob came home from work feeling tired and he wanted to watch the news. The family sat down to supper and were not able to say a word because Bob was watching the news. Bob gulped down his food keeping time with the momentum of the news. He often didn't even know what he was eating. He ate because the food was placed in front of him and it was mealtime. Was he hungry? Or was he tuning in to the clock as an external cue for time to eat? He seemed not to be paying attention to his internal clock (hunger) to regulate the amount of food he ate.

After supper, Bob's wife did the dishes. Bob changed and sometimes helped her dry the dishes. When finished he would turn on the television again to watch his series of evening programmes. As soon as he turned on the television he was hungry again. The association was there between watching television and eating.

Bob had just finished supper. How could he be hungry again? The answer is that he wasn't. Bob never focused on his food while he was eating. He was not tasting and savouring his food. He didn't remember eating, or what he ate.

Perhaps you could exchange the television for the table as a trigger to eat. Try to eat in one place at the table and eat only when you are in that spot. This can help to narrow down one area of the table for eating. Do not play cards or do bookwork or any other activity in that spot. Otherwise, it may trigger you to eat and you will end up building in a new association.

Saving only one spot at the table for eating may be difficult to do and may not be necessary long term. However, for a few weeks it may help you to discover what triggers you to eat. An awareness that there is an association and that you are wasting the calories if you are not tasting and savouring the food, may be all that is necessary to break the habit. After all, you are not depriving yourself when you choose not to eat simply because it is habit. This differs from denying yourself the food when you want it.

For those people living alone, television may provide company. Some people find that by placing a tray in front of the television set while eating, the tray becomes the signal to eat. When they have finished eating, the tray is removed, and the desire is gone. If you use a tray in front of the television set, be conscious of the fact that you are actually tasting your food and savour it slowly. Do not pick up the momentum of the television programme, causing you to eat quickly.

The craving to eat that occurs while you are watching television may come about simply because you need to do something with your hands. If so, try working on a puzzle, do some knitting, or realise that it is all right to do nothing with your hands.

The above situations may cause you to change your behaviour towards food by disassociating it with other activities. However, behaviour change is an external change and may not be natural. A keen awareness of the things that trigger you to eat, and an understanding of the fact that you are not really concentrating on the food enough to eat at a certain time, will help to change your attitude towards these activity/food associations. This internal change in the way that you view these associations can help you to change the way you act towards the food and the activity.

While discussing this in class, Elliot felt that people should have two places to eat, one at the table for the meal and another place specifically for snacks. He discovered that by associating a specific chair with snacks he had to take the trouble to ask the family if he could sit in the specific chair before he could eat.

The process of deciding whether he really wanted to ask them to move out of the specific chair, put a pause into his automatic eating. In many instances he decided that he really wasn't hungry and did not want the food after all. Just as confrontation allows you to put the pause into eating for the sake of eating, or for other reasons, by asking yourself if you are really hungry, confining your eating to only a few places allows you to do the same. It makes you more conscious of whether you are really hungry and allows you to decide if it is psychological or physical hunger. As you begin to develop these skills you eat less because you choose to. It is your decision and you have discovered it so it empowers you to act in a positive way.

When my mother visited from Montreal, she used to come loaded down with all sorts of goodies for our freezer. The association of Mum and home-baked treats came from my growing up in a home where cakes and biscuits were plentiful. It was my Mum's way of saying 'I love you.' This association was so strong that whenever I went back to Montreal or my parents came to Manitoba, I ate too much and I seemed to lose control.

I tried to analyse the situation. Did this occur because I hadn't had these foods for a while and felt deprived? Or was it simply because these foods conjured up nice warm protective feelings of home and Mum? Or was it the association of seeing Mum that made me feel I had to eat these sweets? It probably was a combination of all of these.

Today I am more aware that much of this eating was automatic. I wanted the food, but not the huge quantities I was eating. Tasting and savouring the food and focusing on the food while eating allowed me to be satisfied with less. I got my satisfaction from the first and last few bites.

Because of my lifestyle change, some of the foods Mum brings are too sweet or too rich for me now. So I am satisfied with a taste. My Mum and I had a discussion about this. I love her for herself, not because she bakes these goodies. She may still bring some cakes when she visits, but now they stay in the freezer longer and are not all devoured at once. The balance is there. I don't use them as comfort foods. My walks provide me with all the serenity I need to provide comfort and help me to pace myself better.

The act of eating can cause the release of endorphins which act as a pain reliever and tranquilliser to give you a good feeling. However, the feeling may be only temporary because guilt feelings may occur later about eating the food. Laughter and exercise can also release endorphins that leave you with a good feeling. So go out there and enjoy yourself, and find the fun in physical activity as well.

Some people depend on food more than others do. Cathy could coax Bill to go to Uncle Joe's only by telling him there was food there. Yet his brother, Christopher, was so excited by Uncle Joe's jokes and the fact that Uncle Joe played ball with him. Christopher was more active and slimmer than Bill, who often stayed home with Mum and liked to eat. Because Bill was not as active, food became his source of entertainment. As he grew, so did his waist size. Does food have to be the centre of attention in order for you to have fun?

Every time Jean went to get petrol at a specific garage, she craved a chocolate bar. A few months ago, she bought her favourite brand when she went to pay for the petrol. She continued this a few more times. Had an association built up? What could she do?

She could change garages. The other option would be to recognise the association and to confront it to see if she really wanted the chocolate bar. If she is usually hungry at this time, maybe she could have a snack at afternoon coffee break. She discovered that the chocolate bar didn't really get tasted as it was gulped down quickly. The immediate rise in blood sugar followed by low blood sugar actually caused her to crave more.

Sherry ate a large meal but still wanted dessert. Was this because of psychological hunger or the fact that desserts trigger the end of the meal? If Sherry had been dieting recently, wanting dessert was a natural response to past feelings of deprivation. Try to get away from the diet mentality when you are ordering food in a restaurant. Do you order salad because you believe it is lower in calories and will compensate for the calories in the dessert?

Will salad and dessert keep you going? Depending on the type of salad, it may be high in fat (salad dressing) and contain very little substance in the form of carbohydrate or protein. Check how you feel a few hours later. If dessert triggers the end of the meal, try to find a more suitable replacement. Or is a replacement really necessary as your attitude changes about how to end the meal?

Where it is required, tea with milk serves as a warm ending to the meal. Eat the dessert if you really want it, but if it is simply habit, perhaps you could skip dessert until later and be satisfied with tea. By giving yourself the option to have it later, you are getting rid of the sense of deprivation if you choose not to have it. When you do have the dessert, eat it without guilt. In this way, you will derive more satisfaction from it which will allow you to taste and savour the food better.

By including variety and spontaneity in your day, your life

will become less humdrum and excitement will take its place. Sometimes you may choose to have dessert to signify the end of the meal and sometimes you may choose to have nothing. There is no set rule or perfect way of eating: go with the flow.

EATING OUT

These days people are eating out a lot more and this provides a great opportunity to experience unfamiliar foods and incorporate new ideas into our home cooking. Obviously we have less control over the ingredients that are used in restaurant meals, but the aim is to apply the same approach to eating out as eating in.

Many people binge when eating out. Marilyn used to be very strict with her diet during the week, and looked forward to the weekends when she allowed herself to go off the diet and eat out. Her ritual would be to have no breakfast and maybe no lunch to compensate for the extra calories she consumed at supper. This diet mentality caused her to be overly hungry by supper. She felt starved and therefore overate. She rationalised that it was socially acceptable to binge when eating out.

This starve/binge cycle led to a drop in her metabolic rate. This was her body's way of saying that when she finally did eat, it would 'squirrel away' a little more fat just in case she did something silly again, such as not eating until supper. Marilyn realised that when she went to a restaurant starved, she was not even tasting her food. Marilyn's strategy changed. She ate regularly and went to the restaurant meal pleasantly hungry and enjoyed the food.

Many people eat one way at home and differently when visitors come or when they are at a restaurant. If you choose high-fat foods on these occasions it's no wonder you can't seem to stabilise your weight. There's nothing wrong with eating some foods higher in fat content. But switching back and forth between high-fat and low-fat foods impedes your progress in changing your food preferences.

It's better to discover some low-fat entrées in restaurants that are both physically and psychologically satisfying. Don't feel that you have to bring out the high-fat meals when visitors show up. You can go to any social occasions and be in charge. Keep these principles in mind when you eat out.

Eat Regularly

Eat regular meals during the day. Don't starve at breakfast and lunch to compensate for eating out at supper. This will allow you to feel more energetic throughout the day rather than feeling washed out, waiting for that huge meal to devour at suppertime. You will arrive at the meal pleasantly hungry instead of famished. Being overly hungry leads to quick eating due to the insatiable hunger that you have built up. A pleasant hunger results in enjoying the meal thoroughly, allowing you to feel in charge.

Order What You Really Want

One day, when I was in a restaurant for a meeting around 10:30 a.m., I wanted to eat something. I noticed the cinnamon bread and asked to have it toasted. Forgetting that toasting bread usually means loading it with butter, the result was soggy toast with little texture or cinnamon taste. The lesson I learned was to be assertive. If you are unsure how a food is prepared, ask for it without butter.

If you order what you really want in a restaurant, you feel satisfied. But first you have to tune in to what you really desire. Rose went into the restaurant with her friend and wanted spaghetti and meatballs, which she ordered. She felt satisfied with the meal and it had sustaining power since she satisfied herself both physically and psychologically. By contrast, her friend did not know what she wanted and finally ended up ordering a sandwich. This in itself should have been physically satisfying, yet she wanted more. She had not satisfied the psychological part of her hunger and she craved something more.

You can have what you want in a restaurant so be assertive. One evening Mitchell and I went to a concert and arrived early. We wanted something to drink and went into the cafeteria. We chose fruit juice, a glass of water, and picked up another empty glass. At our seat, we added water to the fruit juice to suit our tastes.

Here is another example. Allison prepared a tasty supper. She ate until she was satisfied and wanted to finish with something chocolate. She and her family decided to go out for a snack. On the dessert menu was ice cream, chocolate brownies, and apple pie. Chocolate brownies were what Allison wanted and she and her friend Grace ordered them. The rest of the family ordered what they wanted.

A few minutes later the waitress came back to say there were no more chocolate brownies. Allison settled for apple pie with ice cream and Grace, after some hesitation, ordered apple pie. But that is not what they really wanted, so why did they order it? Why settle for something that you don't want because you feel you must order something? While they were eating the apple pie, they were still thinking about the chocolate brownies and were still not satisfied, so they wasted those calories.

The next day, Grace, who had a even stronger built-up desire for chocolate, ate several pieces of dark chocolate. Finally she was satisfied. The lesson learned was that refusing the apple pie would probably have yielded the same outcome. She could have bought a chocolate bar at a convenience store instead of having the pie. Decide what you really want and go for it.

If the meal is not enjoyable, you will crave dessert to satisfy that unfulfilled need. For example, the sandwich and chips may be the special of the day. If you do not care for chips, order a salad instead, or order à la carte, perhaps soup and a sandwich.

Try this technique. Say to the waitress, 'I know that the special comes with chips but I would prefer to have the soup so could you arrange this?' The words have special meaning. 'I know,' indicates that you understand the situation. 'But,' states how you feel about the situation. 'So,' is your request for their action.

You can use this form of assertion any time you are in a situation where you need to be direct in a polite manner. If nothing on the menu particularly suits your taste, why not order à la carte? An example of this would be a breakfast of scrambled eggs with dry toast (whole wheat), orange juice, and water. Use the water to dilute the juice as fruit juice is usually strong and too sweet. A substitute for the protein, in this case the egg, would be baked beans on toast.

Use Non-diet Thinking

'I'd better get my fill of the cheesecake now because when I go back on my diet tomorrow I won't be having cheesecake for a while.'

'I feel full but I still have room for a big piece of pie. Afterwards, I'll lie down.'

This diet thinking can be replaced by a more positive attitude.

'I'll take a small piece of that cheesecake. It looks good and I wonder what it tastes like. If I don't try it, I'll be wondering what it tastes like and may end up feeling deprived. This will lead me to binge on whatever is in sight when I get home.'

'I can always have more food later because I feel full now. I can ask the waitress if I can take a piece of pie home for another day when I will appreciate it more. That way I am not denying myself and I am not stuffing myself either.'

When refusing food at a friend's house it's easier to say 'I'm on a diet' because society accepts this reason for denying yourself something you want. If you say you don't want it, it appears to be rude to the hostess. Try saying, 'I'm not hungry right now, maybe later.' Later may or may not come.

Even slim people are often in the diet mentality. Observe different people at a social occasion. Non-dieters, those who are not starving and binging to remain slim, are more selective in their choices. They may eat what they want and may eat a little more than usual, but their regular eating habits prevent them from intentionally binging or overeating.

It is easier to resist food if you are feeling satisfied and realise that this is not the last time that you will see lemon pie for a while. After all, you can buy a pie or make one any time or you can ask to take some home. Slightly undereating at mealtimes to leave room for dessert may be done on special occasions if it is not carried to the extreme.

Eating very little at mealtimes so that you can try all the desserts reverts to the diet mentality. 'I'd better eat all I can now because it may not be there later on.' In a society of plenty, running out of food is not a problem. Non-dieters know this and are more selective in choosing the meal. They will eat desserts only when they truly desire them.

Striving for a Balance of Carbohydrate and Protein

Choose a balance of carbohydrates and protein in your food because you want to, not because you feel you should. You may not always feel like choosing the right balance to give yourself the maximum energy, but striving for this balance and its sustained energy value will result in a satisfying dining-out experience.

Eating in this manner will help you to focus your energy on the mealtime event rather than just the food. The company and entertainment are also part of the evening. Food is no longer the centre of attention for you. You will be able to taste and savour your food and have enough energy to enjoy the rest of the evening. Overeating makes us feel uncomfortable. You don't feel like being sociable and all you want to do is go home and go to bed.

Here are some examples of different restaurants and the kinds of choices that indicate the principle of balance.

ITALIAN

Pasta dishes are great but those with with cream sauces are richer than those served with the traditional tomato sauces and have a higher fat content. The protein content may be minimal. A more balanced option that is lower in fat content is the traditional spaghetti with meat sauce or meatballs You may choose to ask for a tossed salad instead of garlic bread.

Some restaurants skimp on the protein source and give you a hefty portion of noodles topping it off with garlic bread. It is cheaper for the restaurant and customers are usually satisfied since carbohydrates fill you up quickly. However, the insufficient protein content may necessitate a snack later on. Otherwise, insatiable hunger will strike, making you raid the fridge. Decide what you really want. Some cream sauces with sufficient protein content are not too heavy and could be your choice.

FRENCH

French cuisine usually involves a variety of sauces to add flavour to the meat portion of the meal. Try meals cooked in wine sauce rather than in a cream sauce. These meals are tasty and nicely flavoured with herbs. A food doesn't have to be rich to be tasty. For lunch, quiche and salad may be loaded with fat, so take control and minimise the fat by asking for the salad dressing on the side.

CHINESE

The more traditional assortment of deep-fried foods (chicken balls, prawns, etc.) and sweet and sour sauces (spare ribs) have a high-fat content as well as sugar and little meat. There are excellent stir-fried dishes that you can order instead. Ordering one of these with stir-fried Chinese vegetables and the usual rice that comes with the meal presents a colourful and tasty balance. In many cases, you may want to ask for more rice. If you are going with someone else and you choose two different main dishes plus the rice and vegetables, you can still have some variety to the meal. Acquiring a taste for less fattening foods means that you eventually prefer the latter choice to the higher-fat foods.

Ask the waitress when you are unsure if the dish is deep-fried or stir-fried. In one instance, my husband and I ordered a couple of dishes and to our surprise, the chicken dish (lemon chicken) came to us in a deep-fried batter version. We both tried it and didn't care for it. Mitchell picked off the thick batter and ate the little piece of chicken inside. The batter was too greasy for his taste. He shared the rest of my dish and the rice and vegetables and asked the waitress to wrap the rest up for our dog.

GREEK

A variety of kebab dishes (chicken, beef, lamb) served with rice and vegetables offers a nice balance for a meal, lunch or evening.

SALAD BARS

These are often the dieter's choice. Salads certainly fill you up quickly because of the high water content of vegetables, yet salads do not provide the balance you are looking for. Most important of all, is it really what you want to eat or are you eating it simply because you feel it is lower in calories?

Lettuce is relatively low in fibre content but many of the vegetables have a higher fibre content. You get water, vitamins, and minerals but little else. Besides, because of the mayonnaise and cream-based mixtures in salad dishes as well as the dressing itself, the total fat content of a salad can be quite high.

The salad bar choice for a meal can be misleading. Some estimates suggest that selections from a salad bar result in total calorie intake from 250 to 1000 with sixty to seventy percent of these calories coming from fat. It seems to be a healthy selection, but it can lack substance, leading to a binge later because of feelings of deprivation. Bread could accompany this meal to boost the carbohydrate content. Pasta salads may add carbohydrates but may also add to the total fat content.

Eating salads so that you can have dessert is deceiving. In the first place, you may not have saved any calories and certainly not fat content. Furthermore, this thinking puts you right back into the diet mentality. 'I'm having less at lunch so I can have the chocolate mousse.' When you make these kinds of choices, you still end up with very little 'holding-over power' in your meal and this can lead to a binge later on. This may occur because of your lower blood sugar level a few hours later. You are not any further ahead in this situation.

FAST FOODS AND PIZZAS

Ordering a hamburger on an unbuttered bun with a salad can be a nice combination. Try to frequent the restaurants that grill or barbecue rather than fry their hamburgers.

Pizzas can give you carbohydrates from the crust and protein from the cheese and toppings. Go with the thicker crust to increase the carbohydrate content of the meal. Vegetables are often part of the topping. Adding a salad can round out the meal nicely. Some restaurants use the higher-fat cheese which you can notice by the greasy sheen on the pizza, not to mention the greasy feel that it leaves in your mouth. Try different pizza places and food combinations to find the ones that are right for you.

Eating Until Satisfied – the 'Doggy Bag' Option

When eating out you have the option to ask for a doggy bag if you cannot finish your meal. The leftover food may be a treat for lunch the next day. You may also choose to leave what you cannot eat on your plate if you are feeling satisfied and pleasantly full. If suppertime is planned to be later, and you know you will be hungry, schedule a snack for yourself. Stuffing yourself on bread while waiting for your dinner and then forcing the whole dinner down because you paid for it is not truly enjoying the meal.

The snack you ate before the restaurant meal and a little bread at the restaurant will allow you to create the right atmosphere of relaxation so that you are able to eat the meal slowly and enjoy it fully. If you fill up on bread, then you may not have enough room for the meal itself which is really what you are paying for.

Here are some other suggestions that will help to make the restaurant meal what you want it to be.

- Ask for the salad dressing on the side. The house dressing usually contains a nice blend of herbs and may be lower in fat (vinaigrette-based rather than cream-based). If the house dressing is thicker, try dipping salad into dressing. You will end up using less.

- Ask for gravy and sauces to be served on the side or ask for small amounts.

- Ask for butter or sour cream on the side. This allows you to be in control of the quantity that you want. Some potatoes taste so good by themselves that they hardly need any addition of fat to mask or hide the flavour. It's the same for hamburger that is ordered with so many condiments that you do not even taste the hamburger. Or the corn on the cob that is seasoned and loaded with butter and salt. Are you really tasting the corn? You might as well take a bit of butter on the edge of your knife and eat it straight up. The idea of the fat is to enhance not mask the flavour of the food. Decide what you really want by using condiments such as butter, salt, sauces, and gravy tastefully.

- Share your dessert. This will satisfy your curiosity about how it tastes without overstuffing yourself. Be selective and order only what you really want. Substitutions in restaurants are often possible, as long as it isn't the rush hour.

HOW TO ELIMINATE SWINGING ON THE FRIDGE DOOR

- Eat regularly, every three to six hours when physically hungry.
  Purpose Keeps blood sugar from going too low, that could result in insatiable hunger, and frees you from cycles of starvation and binging.

- Eat 'balanced' meals that include carbohydrate and protein at all meals.
  Purpose Stabilises blood sugar, sustains energy, keeps your body in the 'drive' mode.

- Be in charge of food and situations. Use skills of confrontation and distraction techniques to combat 'automatic eating'.
  Purpose Empowers you, freeing you from the obsession of food, recognising that much of your eating is emotional.

- Understand how food affects your body. This allows you to postpone eating certain high-sugar foods on an empty stomach.
  Purpose Prevents your blood sugar from going up quickly, leading to a drop in blood sugar that will make you lose control. Eating a snack if hungry and adding in those 'extras' when your body is better equipped to handle them puts you back in the driver's seat.

- Eat only until satisfied. Learn to tune in to feelings of hunger and feelings of fullness. Allow yourself to be more relaxed with eating. Not feeling guilty allows you to extract more enjoyment from eating. It's permissible to leave something on your plate if you are full.
  Purpose Satisfies your needs by allowing you to eat what you want and at the same time providing you with the skills to realise when your body is saying 'Stop. I'll have more later if I really want it.'

- Put in the 'pause' prior to eating:
  1) By using confrontation and asking yourself if you are really hungry;

  2) By stopping halfway through a meal to consciously reassess if you want more;

  3) By focusing on eating while you are eating, and confining your eating to a minimum number of places so you will think before grabbing something to eat; and

  4) By eating in a relaxed manner, tasting and savouring your food.
  Purpose Helps you find different ways of being more conscious of what you are eating, rather than resorting to 'I see it, I want it' or 'Everyone else is eating, so I'll join the crowd.' You realise that you can participate in the fun and enjoyment without mimicking their every action.

Go with the flow. Gain confidence in your ability. Most of all enjoy the process of discovering or rediscovering yourself.

Tune In to What It Feels Like to Overeat
So you overate. Experience and remember this uncomfortable, heavy feeling and decide whether you like this feeling. Is it allowing you to enjoy the occasion or are you too tired to care? A big meal takes a lot of energy to digest, so the scenario of eating and lying down on the sofa is a common one. Not wanting to repeat this feeling can lead to more instances where you will enjoy the food as well as the event but eat for the enjoyment of it. Eating past the point of satisfaction is often no longer enjoyable.

ACTION POINTS

● Build relaxation into your life.

> Create time for yourself each day.

> Practise deep breathing so that you can use this technique when you need it.

> Create a more relaxed atmosphere in which to eat your food.

> Observe those around you who have the ability to relax easily.

● Plan ahead.

> Pack a breakfast/lunch the night before.

> Have some snacks to hand.

● Recognise triggers to automatic eating and find ways of breaking them. Try eating only at the table for a while and notice the difference. Are you focusing on your food more when you are eating?

● Be assertive.

> Refuse food if you want to.

> Avoid thinking in terms of 'home' and 'restaurant' food. You can eat what you want all the time.

> Ask for sauces to be served separately and take what you want rather than what the chef decides.

13

Gauging Your Progress a Day at a Time

Treat setbacks as a learning experience, a necessary detour towards being the best that you can be!

Make a small change today for a better you tomorrow!

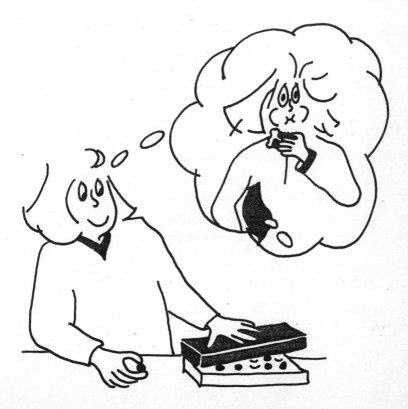

STRESS REDUCTION

Energy comes from a balance in food, activity, and attitude. Too much stress can drain your energy level. Just as you eat and exercise for energy, you can find the stress level that is comfortable and stimulating for you without the feeling of being overwhelmed. Find the balance in your life so that stress can work for you to make you feel alive and vital.

Through the process of self-discovery you can learn how to pull back when the stress level gets above your comfort zone. Here's how to do it.

- By not dieting, you reduce both physical and mental stress.

- By setting yourself free from perfectionism, the 'all-or-nothing' way of thinking that can transfer from food to other areas. If something does not go quite the way you planned, ask yourself what is the worst possible thing that could happen. Could you live with the outcome? This usually puts things in perspective.

Often when the events in your life go wrong another opportunity presents itself. When one door closes, another opens. Be responsive to new ideas. In order to grow, some pain may be involved, yet you will gain a sense of freedom and wisdom, and you will know yourself better. Growth can be inspirational.

Consider these points in your daily routine. Enjoy activity as a release valve so that you exercise for fun. Even if it's hard to get going, if you tune into your body's needs the benefits of vitality and feeling good about yourself gained from physical activity will keep you going. Remember that action creates momentum.

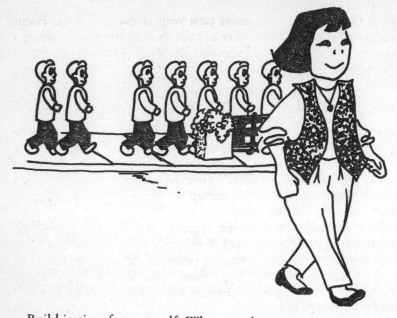

Build in time for yourself. When you have put that pause into your day you have time to catch your breath and enjoy life, rather than let it pass you by. Assess and evaluate your own situation. Practise some relaxation techniques such as deep breathing. This helps you to unwind. Too much stress can drain energy even if you are eating in a healthy manner and exercising regularly.

Like yourself and accept yourself the way you are. This does not mean that you won't do anything to try to improve yourself. It means that you care enough about yourself to nurture yourself and take care of your body and mind. Be the best that you can be!

Allow yourself to be you. Release yourself from attaching your self-worth to the number on the scale, to compliments or criticism, or to what you look like. Unlock the little child in you. As people grow older they tend to become more serious and are bogged down with a planned and organised life. Restore some spontaneity and fun in your routine to keep you interested and vital. Lighten up! Relax!

Believe in yourself and have the confidence in your own ability to accomplish goals by using such assertiveness in everyday life situations. By confronting situations and dealing with them you will not move past your stress level zone. Focus on your progress. The ability to take things calmly can diffuse a potentially difficult and explosive situation. Be proactive rather than reactive.

BELIEFS AND ATTITUDES AFFECT EXPECTATIONS

If you need praise to feel good about yourself you may feel badly if you do not receive it. Self-doubt may set in. Remember the affirmation: 'I like myself. I am a worthwhile person, no matter what anyone says or does.' Turn your negative feelings into something positive. Catch yourself when you put yourself down and praise yourself instead.

Rather than feel defeated, accept setbacks as part of the growing process. If you feel that you can do it, you can. The inner strength you gain from a positive attitude will translate into the ability to get things done. Accept that some things cannot be changed and stop trying to change them. Be satisfied with the things you can do.

Enjoy the journey instead of focusing only on the destination. Focusing on the process rather than the end result reduces the stress level and you will, with time, reach your goal.

A DAY AT A TIME

Small accomplishments in lifestyle changes can be compared to building a wall one brick at a time. Once you begin to make lifestyle changes the wall will begin to become stronger, making it more difficult to knock down. Don't be discouraged by temporary setbacks. They are part of the growth process. Don't forget that Edison had about 2000 temporary setbacks before the light bulb got invented.

Success is an ongoing process. It is the daily expression, acceptance, and appreciation of yourself. Each time you achieve a mini-goal and make a lifestyle change more permanent, you feel good and your self-esteem goes up. The life process itself is ninety-five percent of the fun and one hundred percent of the reward. Using your energy to point your life in the right direction will help you to learn, practise, and enjoy your way to better health. This is your lifetime goal.

In their book *Your Vitality Quotient*,[1] Earle and Imrie used the analogy of an archer to describe this life direction. You are not so much focusing on the end result of aiming at the target as on becoming at one with the process of drawing the bow and releasing the arrow. You are the flight of the arrow. The bonus is that when you truly focus on the process, you inevitably hit the bull's-eye. The difference in this way of thinking is that your energy is focused on the process itself (i.e. lifestyle changes) rather than solely on the end result (i.e. numbers on the scale).

Redefining success in terms of lifestyle changes and health status rather than the tangible result of weight loss puts a new perspective on how you feel about your weight. What does success mean to you? In the past it may have been defined as weight loss visible on the scale. Chances are this success was not long term. Why not try for something more permanent?

Keep in mind that with rare exceptions, none of the available programmes for treating obesity are based on current scientific knowledge. If they were, according to Wayne Callaway, Associate Clinical Professor of Medicine at George Washington University, these programmes could not promise rapid weight loss.[2] It seems we have been using an inaccurate and ineffective measuring tool to judge long-term success.

THE THREE Ps TO LONG-TERM SUCCESS

The internal changes made by lifestyle changes motivate people to keep practising those lifestyle changes. This fresh approach to health is characterised by the three Ps.

Perspective
With a positive perspective on life, you learn to be more flexible, accept life's highs and lows, and learn from them. You no longer isolate specific instances and blame others or yourself for shortcomings; you put the problem into proper perspective. This new lease on life gives you the opportunity to savour the precious moments and deal with the 'downs' as stepping stones to something better. It is part of the plan to mould you into reaching your full potential in health and in life. Breathing new

excitement into life allows you to take on new challenges and strive to be the best that you can be in every aspect of life!

Priority

With the new attitude that you have learned, you need to take time for yourself and make this a priority. We know that you have the choice to keep your life in balance or to be overwhelmed with your unending list of duties and responses to external cues. Feeling better about yourself and having confidence in your ability minimises the effect that comments from others have on you.

When you set your priorities and schedule 'time off' for yourself, you leave some time for unexpected emergencies. Improving your self-esteem shows you that you do not have to answer to anyone else but yourself. There will always be those who try to sabotage your best efforts or make you feel insignificant. You have learned to put this in the proper perspective. The final decision is yours.

With an improved self-image you no longer need as many compliments to prove yourself to others. It no longer matters to you what others think. You strive for excellence in the best way that you know how and you realise that the struggle for perfection is not worth the effort. Perhaps it is superficial, artificial, and energy-draining rather than a constructive, meaningful experience contributing to your growth.

Perseverance

'Hanging in there' is certainly worth the effort. The result is a new lifestyle that puts your life in balance and gives you an inner glow that radiates outward and brings with it health and vibrancy. You have a sense of accomplishment. This way of life is one of celebration and it is for a lifetime; it doesn't end when you attain a temporary goal.

The key to keeping lifestyle change going is to enjoy the process. Just as a flower buds, and only with time does it come into full bloom, so your process of growth will also be gradual. You could take the time to note the more positive ways that you are dealing with situations, and savour the freedom to live your life to the fullest.

SUCCESS REDEFINED

One source of stress in people's lives is that they don't feel good about themselves and they lack self-esteem. They have a lot of anxiety. They feel they're 'losing it'. By redefining success as the process of improving your health and lifestyle, your physical and mental stress is reduced. Consider these points.

● Feel 'in charge'.

● Feel good about yourself; improve your self-image and gain more confidence.

● Increase your activity gradually and enjoy it.

● Make gradual lifestyle changes because you want to.

● As your waist/hip ratio improves it indicates a lower risk of heart disease, high blood pressure, and diabetes.

● Simplify your lifestyle for healthier living.

● Celebrate food in its proper place. Food is no longer the centre of life.

● Look forward to getting up in the morning.

● Feel free to eat.

Overall, the above points define an improved health status. Healthier individuals in both body and mind are more apt to reach their full potential, which makes life fuller at every moment.

RATE YOUR PROGRESS IN THE PROCESS OF HEALTHY LIVING

Complete the Lifestyle Quiz again on p287 and compare this evaluation to the assessment you made at the beginning of the book. Note where your greatest improvement in lifestyle behaviour occurred. Use the checklist on p289 to pinpoint areas that need more focus to achieve your new lifestyle. Focus on your improvement in attitude and lifestyle change.

LIFESTYLE QUIZ

1 Always
2 Very often
3 Often
4 Sometimes
5 Rarely
6 Never

☐ I am unhappy with myself the way I am.

☐ I am preoccupied with a desire to be thinner.

☐ I weigh myself several times a week.

☐ I am more concerned with the number on the scale than my overall sense of wellbeing.

☐ I think about burning up calories when I exercise.

☐ I am out of tune with my body for natural signs of hunger and fullness.

☐ I eat for reasons other than physical hunger.

☐ I eat too quickly, not taking time to focus on my meal and to taste, savour, and enjoy my food.

☐ I fail to take time for activities for myself.

☐ I fluctuate between periods of sensible, nutritious eating and out-of-control eating.

☐ I give too much time and thought to food.

☐ I tend to skip meals, especially early in the day, so I can 'save up' my food for one big feast.

☐ I engage in all-or-nothing thinking. I tend to feel that if I can't do it all, or do it well, what's the point?

☐ I try to be all things to all people.

☐ I strive for perfection in my life.

☐ I criticise myself for not achieving my goals.

☐ **Total** Add 4 to the score to determine your percentage.

Please share your success with others

Now that you've discovered the true benefits of healthy living and size acceptance, you can help spread the message.

Your assistance is important. Our programmes are fine-tuned through the research data that is requested in the lifestyle quizzes. Your response to these questions is the key to the process. Total professional confidentiality is assured, and your reward is the satisfaction of knowing that YCCD will be more effective and have broader appeal.

How to participate
1. Make a photocopy of your beginning quiz (p8).

2. Make a photocopy of the concluding quiz (p287).

3. Now that you have worked through the book and made adjustments to your lifestyle and attitude, there will undoubtedly be a change in your response to these same questions. Mentally celebrate your new score!

4. Complete the postal address information below.

5. Send your photocopies and address to the HUGS™ office at **Hugs International Inc., Box 102A, RR#3 Portage la Prairie, Manitoba, Canada R1N 3A3.** or FAX (204)428-5072.

6. In appreciation of your participation we'll provide you with two complimentary issues of the HUGS™ newsletter – a bi-annual publication full of healthy living inspiration and ongoing practical help ideas.

NAME

ADDRESS

TOWN   COUNTY   POSTAL CODE

HOME PHONE   WORK PHONE

THE YCCD HEALTHY LIVING CYCLE
**It begins with self-acceptance,
simply feeling good about yourself.**

As you follow our healthy living steps, your physical and mental
wellbeing will be constantly improving.

Chapter 2
Throw the scales away and focus on rebuilding health.

Chapter 3
Exercise regularly at your own level with an activity you enjoy.

Chapter 4
Balance your meals appropriately to fill your needs for fullness and energy.

Chapter 4
Eat regularly starting with a balanced breakfast.

Chapter 5
Be creative in food preparation using herbs and spices to replace fatty
ingredients.

Chapter 6
Tune in to your natural hunger signals. Eat whatever you want whenever you
want, as long as you are physically hungry.

Chapter 7
Eat until you are physically satisfied, and not overly full.

Chapter 8
Focus on the internal rewards of energy and wellbeing.

Chapter 9
Use skills of confrontation to cope with bursts of psychological hunger.

Chapter 9
STOP, TASTE, SAVOUR and ENJOY your food to the fullest.

Chapter 10
Exercise your choice in the purchase of products suited to your new tastes.

Chapter 11
Ensure you are hungry, not merely thirsty.

Chapter 12
Take time for yourself and relax. You are special too!

Chapter 13
Treat setbacks as a learning experience, a necessary detour towards being the
best that you can be!

Chapter 13
Make a small change today for a better you tomorrow!

BE THE BEST THAT YOU CAN BE!

ACTION POINTS

- Attach your self-worth to who you are and what you do.

- Take things slowly – one day at a time.

- Treat setbacks as learning experiences.

- Make a small change today for a healthier you tomorrow.

- Remember: **you count, calories don't!**

Looking ahead

If your main goal as you came into the YCCD programme was to lose weight, but you have not yet lost any weight, perhaps the goal has to be looked at again. If you remember, we said a goal of weight loss does not achieve health and permanent lifestyle change. Focusing on a goal of weight loss shifts the emphasis from lifestyle habits that are integral in stabilising and maintaining any weight lost. Remember that fluctuations in body weight are more harmful to health than if you stabilise at a higher weight.

We all make decisions that affect the rest of our lives. We can choose to take responsibility for them and move on or continue to dwell on the past causing more stress and unhappiness which leads to more eating. In this way, the process of healthy living is no longer natural but forced. The journey is no longer enjoyable. Rather the destination becomes foremost in your mind.

It's your choice – continue to recognise and accept the internal benefits gained and strive for unconditional self-acceptance, or go back on the bandwagon that brings with it irritability, preoccupation with weight and food, and even larger body size a few years later.

Diets don't work. The greatest chance to reach your health potential is through healthy living. Why give up that chance now that you have come so far? Lifestyle change doesn't happen overnight. If it did it would simply be another diet under the new banner 'lifestyle'.

HOW FAR HAVE YOU PROGRESSED?

- Have you cultivated a preference for lower fat foods?

- Have you cultivated a preference for less sugary foods?

- Are you starting to enjoy incorporating more activity into your lifestyle?

- Are you dealing with why you are eating in the first place?
- Are you using confrontation to really determine if you want certain foods?
- Are you making small changes to build in some time for yourself?
- Are you thinking like a non-dieter?

Every yes answer is a success!

When you can answer yes to all these lifestyle shifts, physical changes might take place. If you rush this process, you will certainly end up back in the diet mentality. The more you have dieted and the older you are, the longer it will take to make the new process enjoyable. But if it's pleasurable and you have an attitude of self-discovery and experimentation, it really doesn't matter how long the new process takes. If you allow changes to take place over a five-year period, your body will readjust to its natural weight comfortably, and will maintain it. No matter what the outcome, you are to be congratulated on taking this road. This is the way you will be healthier and happier.

Your success brings renewed confidence and self-acceptance, energy, enjoyment of increased activity, feeling better about yourself, and improved eating habits.

Our international network of over eighty licensed facilitators in five countries is growing. Contacts for the You Count, Calories Don't (HUGS) programme worldwide are:

UK and Ireland:

Mary Evans Young
Diet Breakers
Barford St Michael
Banbury
Oxon OX15 0UA
Fax: 01869 337177

Canada and USA:

Linda Omichinski
HUGS International Inc.
Box 102A RR#3
Portage la Prairie, MB
Canada R1N 3A3
Fax: (204) 428 5072

YOU COUNT, Calories Don't Programme and Facilitator Kit

Our integrated plan for lifelong better health is at the forefront of the non-diet movement. Many people's situations require some type of lifestyle adjustment to modify health risk. This is where the YOU COUNT, Calories Don't programme fits in.

The programme focuses on health and self-acceptance rather than dieting and weight loss. By instilling new and positive attitudes about food and physical activity, the programme moves individuals from preoccupation around food, weight, and behaviour (the insidious diet mentality) to a feeling of empowerment and self-reliance. With confidence and newly acquired skills, individuals accomplish a gradual lifestyle shift that maximises full health potential.

The programme is delivered in a ten-weekly workshop format that includes group discussion and participation, attitudinal analysis methods, and nutritional education.

To join the growing international network of licensed Facilitators (health professionals, personnel officers, counsellors, teachers etc.) delivering the YCCD programme contact:

MARY EVANS YOUNG in England
or LINDA OMICHINSKI in Canada
address and telephone numbers on previous page

Here is what some Facilitators have already said:

- the programme is brilliant;
- it's easy to use, easy to follow;
- comprehensive, very complete;
- high-quality material;
- puts my thinking into practice;
- it's all there!

Notes

NOTES FOR PREFACE

1. *University of California, Berkeley Wellness Letter*, 'Great bodies come in many shapes', Vol. 7, issue 5, Feb. 1991.
2. Joe McVoy, PhD, 'Treatment: New directions needed for 1990s', *Obesity & Health*, Vol. 5, No. 6, Nov./Dec. 1991.
3. 'Obesity: Year 2000 crisis?, *Obesity & Health*, Vol. 5, No. 5, Sept./Oct. 1991.
4. Donna Ciliska and Carla Rice, 'Body Image/Body Politics', *Healthsharing*, Summer, 1989.

NOTES FOR INTRODUCTION

1. S.C. Wooley, PhD, and O.W. Wayne Wooley, PhD, 'Thinness Mania', *American Health*, October, 1986.
2. S.C. Wooley, PhD, and O.W. Wooley, PhD, 'Should obesity be treated at all?', *Eating and its disorders*, Stunkard, A.J., and Stellar, E. editors, New York, 1984.

NOTES FOR CHAPTER 1

1. *Nutrition Forum*, Jan. 1988.
2. *University of California Berkeley Wellness Letter*, Vol. 7, No. 5, Feb. 1991.
3. *Nutrition News*, Winter 1990.
4. *International Obesity Newsletter*, Vol. 2, No. 9, Sept. 1988.
5. *Ann. Intern. Med.*, Dec. 1985, pp1006–1009.
6. *Mayo Clinic Nutrition Letter*, Vol. 2, No. 7, July 1989.
7. *Dairy Council Digest*, Vol. 59, No. 3, May/June, 1988.
8. *University of California, Berkeley Wellness Letter*, Vol. 4, No. 12, Sept. 1988.
9. Kevin Anderson, PhD, Framingham Study; Dr W.B. Kannel, Boston University of Medicine.
10. Dr George Christakis, 'The Effect of Dietary Cholesterol on Serum Cholesterol: An Interpretive Review', Adjunct Professor of Nutrition, University of Miami, School of Medicine, Miami, Florida.

11. *Dairy Council Digest*, Vol. 58, No. 5, Sept./Oct. 1987.
12. *Harvard Medical School Health Letter*, Nov. 1987.
13. *Dairy Council Digest*, Jan./Feb. 1988.
14. Macdonald, CDA Conf., 1988.
15. *New England Journal of Medicine* 322: 147, 1990.
16. *Nutrition & the M.D.*, Vol. 15, No. 1, Jan. 1989.
17. *University of California, Berkeley Wellness Letter,* Vol. 6, issue 1, Oct. 1989.
18. *New England Journal of Medicine* 1991:324:1839–44, taken from *Obesity & Health*, 'Yo-yo dieting threatens heart. Gain-lose-gain cycle may be as risky as staying obese', Vol. 5, No. 6, Nov./Dec. 1991.
19. *Int J Obesity* 14: 303, 1990.
20. *Nutrition & the M.D.*, July 1990.
21. Dr Steven L. Shumak, M.D., F.R.C.P.(C), 'Deterioration of Glucose Control in NIDDM', *Canadian Diabetes*, Vol. 4, No. 2, June 1991.
22. Dr Coopan, 'Special report on Type II diabetes', *Joslin* magazine, Fall, 1986.
23. *Diabetes Education Resource Manual*, Winnipeg, MB, 1986.
24. Sandi Meredith R.P. Dt., Lawrence A. Leiter M.D., F.R.C.P.(C), F.A.C.P., Loren D. Grossman, M.D., F.R.C.P.(C), 'Commercial Weight Loss Clinics in the Treatment of Obese Patients with Diabetes: Are They Safe?', *Canadian Diabetes*, Vol. 4, No. 1, March 1991.

NOTES FOR CHAPTER 2

1. Dr Frank Katch, Nutrition and Life-style, Kellogg Symposium, 1988.
2. Dorice M. Czajka-Narins, PhD, and Ellen Parham, PhD, R.D., 'Fear of Fat: Attitudes toward Obesity – The Thinning of America', *Nutrition Today*, Jan./Feb. 1990.
3. *Nutrition & the M.D.*, 'Changing Body Fat Patterns', Vol. 14, No. 11, Nov. 1988.
4. Cheryl Jennings-Sauer, M.A., R.D., L.D., *Living Lean by Choosing More*, Taylor Publishing Co., 1989.
5. *Obesity and Health Newsletter*, Vol. 4, No. 6, June 1990.
6. *Obesity & Health*, 'The world of weight loss fraud', Vol. 4, No. 9, Sept. 1990.
7. *Ann Intern Med* 99:14, 1983 taken from *Nutrition & the M.D.*, Aug. 1990.
8. S.C. Wooley and O.W. Wooley, 'Obesity and Women – I. A Closer Look at the Facts', *Women's Studies Int. Quart.*, Vol. 2, Pergamon Press Ltd., pp 69–79, 1979.
9. *Nutrition & the M.D.*, Vol. 16, No. 7, July 1990.
10. *Am J Clin Nutr* 49:1105, 1989.
11. *Am Intern Med* 103:994, 1985.
12. *New England Journal of Medicine* 1991:324:1839–44, taken from *Obesity & Health*, 'Yo-yo dieting threatens heart. Gain-lose-gain cycle may be as risky as staying obese', Vol. 5, No. 6, Nov./Dec. 1991.

13. *Int J Obesity* 14:303, 1990.
14. Ibid ref. 11.
15. *New England Journal of Medicine* 1991:324:1839–44; taken from *Obesity & Health*, Vol. 5, No. 6, Nov./Dec. 1991, 'Yo-yo dieting threatens heart. Gain-lose-gain cycle may be as risky as staying obese.'
16. Linda J. McCargar, PhD, R.D.N., and Helen Yeung, BSc, R.D.N., 'The Effects of Weight Cycling on Metabolism and Health', *Can. Diet. Assoc.* 52:101–106, 1991.
17. *University of California, Berkeley Wellness Letter*, Vol. 7, issue 1, Oct. 1990.
18. *Dairy Council Digest*, Vol. 59, No. 3, May/June, 1988.
19. C. Brown and D. Forgay, 'An Uncertain Well-Being: Weight Control and Self Control', *Healthsharing*, Winter: 11–15, 1987.
20. William Bennett and Joel Gurin, *The Dieter's Dilemma*, Basic Books, New York, May, 1982.
21. *Harvard Medical School Health Letter*, 'It's the Butter, not the Bread', Vol. 13, No. 9, July 1988.
22. *J Clin Invest* 76: 1019, 1985.
23. *J Clin Invest* 64: 1336, 1979.
24. *National Institute of Nutrition*, 'Metabolic Consequences of Weight-Reduction Diets', Review No. 6, July 1988.
25. Ellen Parham, PhD, R.D., 'Alternative goals render successful outcomes likely', *Obesity & Health*, Vol. 5, No. 4, July/Aug. 1991.
26. *Dairy Council Digest*, Mar./Apr. 1985, published by National Dairy Council.
27. *Dairy Council Digest*, Vol. 62, No. 2, Mar./Apr. 1991.
28. F.W. Ashley, W.B. Kannel. 'Relation of weight change to changes in atherogenic traits: The Framingham Study', *J Chronic Dis* 27:103–114, 1974.
29. Kelly Brownell, 'American Health and Obesity and Weight Control: The Good And Bad of Dieting', *Nutrition Today*, May/June 1987.
30. *Obesity & Health Newsletter*, Vol. 5, No. 4, July/August 1991.

NOTES FOR CHAPTER 3

1. *Nutrition & the M.D.*, Nov. 1990.
2. *Sports Medicine* 1:446, 1984.
3. *University of California, Berkeley Wellness Letter*, Oct. 1990.
4. National Institute of Nutrition, *Rapport*, 'Effective Energy Content of Fat', Vol. 2, No. 3, July 1987.
5. Kathy King Helm, R.D., 'Sports Nutrition Basics', *Nutrition Forum*, Vol. 5, No. 6, July/Aug, 1988.
6. *Member's Magazine*, Participation Network, Vol. 3, No. 1, Winter, 1986.
7. Ibid. ref. No. 5.
8. J.P. Flatt, 'Dietary fat, carbohydrate balance, and weight maintenance; effects', *Am J Clin Nutr* 45: 296, 1987.

9. Faulkner, International Conference on Exercise, Fitness, and Health, Toronto, 1988.
10. *Dairy Council Digest*, Vol 60, No. 4, July/Aug. 1989. Published by National Dairy Council, 6300 North River Road, Rosemont, Il. 60018-4233.
11. Greenwood, M.R.C. (Ed.), *Obesity: Contemporary Nutrition*, New York: Churchill Livingstone, 1983.
12. *University of California, Berkeley Wellness Letter*, Vol. 5, No. 7, April 1989.
13. *University of California, Berkeley Wellness Letter*, Oct. 1990.
14. Ibid. ref. No. 5.
15. *Nutrition & the M.D.*, 'Exercise and Metabolic Rate, Diet Therapy/ Obesity Update', Feb. 1988.
16. Health & Welfare Canada's *New Guidelines for Healthy Eating*, 1991.
17. James O. Hill, PhD; Phillip B. Sparling, EdD; Toni W. Shields, MS; and Patricia A. Heller, R.D., 'Effects of exercise and food restriction on body composition and metabolic rate in obese women', *Am J Clin Nutr* 46: 622–30, 1987.
18. Lindsey C. Henson, M.D., PhD; David C. Poole, PhD; Clyde P. Donahoe, PhD; and David Heber, M.D., PhD, 'Effects of exercise training on resting energy expenditure during caloric restriction', *Am J Clin Nutr* 46: 893–9.
19. Ibid ref. No. 9.
20. Paffenbarger et al, of Harvard Alumni. *Diabetes Care*, Vol. 13, No. 2, Feb. 1990.
21. 'Exercise & Renal Stone Formation, Diet Therapy/Obesity Update', *Nutrition & the M.D.* Feb. 1988.
22. *University of California, Berkeley Wellness Letter*, Vol. 5, No. 3, Dec. 1988.
23. *University of California, Berkeley Wellness Letter*, Vol. 6, issue 4, Jan. 1990.
24. *University of California, Berkeley Wellness Letter*, Vol. 7, issue 5, Feb. 1991.

NOTES FOR CHAPTER 4

1. *Lancet* 2:614, 1964.
2. Obesity and Weight Control, Aspen, 1988.
3. Ibid.
4. Dr Wayne Callaway, Kellogg Nutrition Symposium, Toronto, April, 1988.
5. N. Theresa Glanville, PhD, 'Central Nervous System Regulation of Food Intake: the Role of Dietary Signals', *J Can. Diet. Assoc.*, Vol. 50, No. 3, Summer, 1989.
6. Barbara J. Rolls, Marion Hetherington, and Victoria J. Burley, 'The Specificity of Satiety: The Influence of Foods of Different Macronutrient Content on the Development of Satiety', *Psychology & Behavior*, Vol. 43, pp 145–153, Pergamon Press, 1988.
7. *University of California, Berkeley Wellness Letter*, Nov. 1988.

8. *Am J Clin Nutr* 45: 323, 1987. Article taken from *Nutrition & the M.D.*, Vol. 16, No. 3, March 1990.
9. *University of California, Berkeley Wellness Letter*, June 1991.
10. Ibid.
11. D.J.A. Jenkins, T.M.S. Wolever, R.H. Taylor, et al., 'Glycemic Index of foods: a physiological basis for carbohydrate exchange', *Am J Clin Nutr* 34: 362–6, 1981. (Data obtained from normal individuals.)
12. F. Xavier Pi-Sunyer, M.D., 'Fiber: What's in it for You?', *Diabetes Forecast*, May/June, 1983.
13. *Protect Yourself*, Nov. 1987.

NOTES FOR CHAPTER 5

1. *Dairy Council Digest*, July/August 1988.
2. *University of California, Berkeley Wellness Letter*, Vol. 5, No. 1, Oct. 1988.
3. *National Institute of Nutrition*, July 1988.
4. *Harvard Medical School Health Letter*, July 1988.
5. Beef Information Centre News Release, March 4, 1987.
6. *Obesity & Health*, July/August 1991.
7. *International Journal of Obesity*, 17:237, 1993.
8. L. Omichinski and H. Wiebe Hildebrand, *Tailoring Your Tastes*, TAMOS Books Inc., Manitoba, 1995.
9. Ibid.
10. Ibid.

NOTES FOR CHAPTER 6

1. Janet Polivy and Peter Herman, *Breaking the Diet Habit*. Basic Books, New York, 1983.

NOTES FOR CHAPTER 9

1. *ESHA Research*, Spring 1991.

NOTES FOR CHAPTER 10

1. *University of California, Berkeley Wellness Letter*, Vol. 5, No. 3, Dec. 1988.

NOTES FOR CHAPTER 11

1. A.B. Natow, J. Heslin, *Geriatric Nutrition*, Boston, Mass. 1980:192.
2. *University of California, Berkeley Wellness Letter*, June 1991.

3. *University of California, Berkeley Wellness Letter*, June 1991.
4. *Am J Clin Nutr* 37: March 1983, pp 416–420.
5. *Mayo Clinic Nutrition Letter*, Feb. 1990.
6. *National Institute of Nutrition Review*, No. 2, May 1987.

NOTES FOR CHAPTER 13

1. Richard Earle, *Your Vitality Quotient*, Random House, Mississauga, Ontario, 1989.
2. *Obesity and Health Journal*, Vol. 4, No. 6, June 1990.

Further Reading

GENERAL

Shelley Bovey, *The Forbidden Body*, Pandora Press, London, 1994

Mary Evans Young, *Diet Breaking, having it all without having to diet*, Hodder & Stoughton, London, 1995

Tom Sanders and Peter Bazalgette, *You Don't Have to Diet*, Bantam, London, 1994

Yes! (Leading bi-monthly magazine offering a positive approach to life and health for women size 16+. Available from newsagents.)

Db (Diet Breakers' own magazine. See Order Form page)

FOR HEALTH PROFESSIONALS INTERESTED IN THE GROWING MOVEMENT FOR HEALTH AND SELF-ACCEPTANCE

Obesity and Health Journal. Healthy Living Institute, Route 2, Box 905, Hettinger, N.D. 58639. Telephone 1(701)567-2845. (An excellent journal containing very progressive articles and research findings.)

Donna Ciliska, R.N., Ph.D., *Beyond Dieting: Psychoeducational Interventions for Chronically Obese Women: A Non-Dieting Approach*, Brunner/Mazel, Inc., 119 Union Square West, New York, New York 10003, 1990. Toll free 1-800-363-2845. (Excellent research in this area.)

Association for Health Enrichment of Large People (AHELP), P.O. Drawer C, Radford, Virginia 24143. FAX 1(703)633-1767; for information call Joe McVoy, Ph.D., St Albans Psychiatric Hospital, 1-800-368-3468 US or 1(703)633-4501. (Ask for AHELP brochure. Most leaders in this movement belong to this progressive organisation.)

David M. Garner, Ph.D., and Susan C. Wooley, Ph.D., 'Confronting the Failure of Behavioral and Dietary Treatments for Obesity', *Clinical Psychology Review*, Vol. 11, pp 729–80, 1991. (An excellent review article substantiating this approach.)

Index

Order Form
Resources for the non-diet lifestyle

☐ **You Count, Calories Don't Audio Tapes**
Stop dieting and start living. Set of three tapes provides new perspectives on life, leading to increased confidence about making decisions that are best for your situation. Learn how to use positive language, relax, and be more assertive as you take your focus off weight.
£19.95 including post & packing. UK and Ireland only.

☐ **You Count, Calories Don't Fitness Video**
Gentle, physical activity. If other exercise tapes have left you feeling that fitness is not for you, you'll appreciate our gentle and fun approach to activity. Relaxed participants have been filmed in a natural, outdoor setting. You can enjoy moving at a level that leaves you feeling energised, not exhausted. Experience our refreshing new approach. Gain the desire to be more active.
£9.95 plus £2 post and packing.

☐ **Diet Breaking, having it all without having to diet**
Important and inspiring book by the founder of Diet Breakers, Mary Evans Young.
£6.99 plus £1 post and packing. Also available from Hodder and Stoughton Publishers, Bookpoint, 39 Milton Park, Abingdon, Oxon OX14 4BR. Please make cheques payable to Hodder Headline PLC.

☐ **Db**
Leading high-quality magazine covering news, health information, advice, lifestyle, fashion, gossip, and humour to support the non-diet, healthier way of living.
Annual Subscription: £10 for five issues, includes membership to Diet Breakers.
Please add £5 if outside UK or Ireland.

☐ **Postcards**
Humorous postcards that make a point and spread the anti-diet message. Two of each: **How to lose money** and **Don't change your body, change the rules.**
Four for £1, please send medium SAE with order.

☐ **The Health Risks of Weight Loss**
An authoritative report by Professor Frances Berg, Editor of *Healthy Weight Journal*, bringing together international research on the effects of dieting.
£15 including post & packing.

☐ **You Don't Have to Diet**
A 'must' for anyone wanting to ditch the diet mentality. By Professor Tom Sanders, one of Britain's leading nutritionists, and Peter Bazalgette.
£5.99 plus £1 post and packing.

Diet Breakers' Healthy Lifestyle Booklet – provides guidance and support for non-dieters and includes details of our courses and workshops. £1 plus 25p postage and packing.

I would like to purchase the resources ticked above.

Name ....

Address ....

....

....

Telephone (h)............................... (w) ....

Please make chq./p.o. payable to Diet Breakers for £..... and send to DIET BREAKERS, Barford St Michael, Banbury, OX15 0UA.

Order Form

ADDITIONAL RESOURCES

☐ **Teens & Diets – No Weigh:** Building the road to healthier living. Information package $5. A new programme aiming to prevent the onset of a diet lifestyle and build healthier living patterns. Emphasizes skill building around self-esteem, assertiveness, critical thinking, hands-on cooking, nondiet nutrition concepts and physical activity.

☐ *HUGS Audio Tapes** set $41.95 (including daily affirmation plan for lifelong better health) plus shipping air $10; surface $5
Stop dieting and start living. Set of three tapes provides new perspectives on life leading to increased confidence about making decisions that are best for your situation. Learn how to use positive language, relax, and be more assertive as you take your focus off weight.

☐ *HUGS Club News* Annual subscription (four issues) Canada $15 (Can$) plus GST; USA $15 (US$); Overseas $25 (Can$)
Includes group discussion features. A support network of news, articles, inspiration, and motivation designed to keep the reader off the diet roller coaster and linked with others who have chosen the non-diet lifestyle.

☐ *HUGS Journal Analysis* Seven-day analysis $60
A personal counselling session. Find out how your activity and eating are affecting your energy levels and outlook on life.

☐ *HUGS at Home* $199 (includes indexed binder guide, **You Count, Calories Don't**, Tailoring Your Tastes & Audio Tapes, HUGS Club News subscription, and a Journal Analysis) plus shipping air $30; surface $150
Here's the answer when HUGS classes aren't available in your area.

☐ *HUGS Facilitator Kit* for programme delivery. Complete information package $10. Our international network of licensees is growing constantly. The information package explains the HUGS approach and how HUGS resources can be used in the community, in fitness facilities, in hospitals, in clinics, in workplaces, and in educational institutions. HUGS self-training kit equips the facilitator to deliver cost recovery programmes and/or develop an independent business.

☐ **Tailoring Your Tastes** ea $19.95 (Can$); $14.95 (US$) + shipping air $20; surface $10
A companion to You Count, Calories Don't this innovative concept cookbook emphasizes a convenient 3-step process to changing recipes from which you can adapt your own favourites recipes. A useful resource for anyone wanting to learn how to tailor their tastes to appreciate the tastes and textures of healthier foods.

☐ **I'd like to purchase the resources ticked above.**

Name...

Street address...................................

City, Prov/State.................................

Postal Code/Zip.................................

Phone (H)......................(W)............

Fax...

Cheque enclosed ☐

Visa No. ....

Mastercard No.................................

Expiry date........... Signature................

Total Cost (all items) ....

Shipping Charges ....

GST (Canada) ....

Total $ ....

Please send this form with payment to:

HUGS International Inc.
Box 102A, RR#3
Portage la Prairie, MB
Canada R1N 3A3

E mail lomichin@portage.net

Fax orders
001 204 428 5072

BECOME A LICENSED FACILITATOR

Interested in becoming a licensed facilitator? Contact Mary Evans Young at Diet Breakers if you live in the UK or Irealand and Linda Omichinski at HUGS if you live elsewhere.